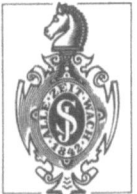

Secretion and Action of Gonadotropins

Physiology and Clinic

Edited by
B. Runnebaum T. Rabe L. Kiesel W. E. Merz

With 51 Figures

Springer-Verlag Berlin Heidelberg GmbH 1984

Professor Dr. med. BENNO RUNNEBAUM
Universitäts-Frauenklinik
Abteilung Gynäkologische Endokrinologie
Voßstraße 9
D-6900 Heidelberg 1

Dr. med. THOMAS RABE
Universitäts-Frauenklinik
Abteilung Gynäkologische Endokrinologie
Voßstraße 9
D-6900 Heidelberg 1

Dr. med. LUDWIG KIESEL
Universitäts-Frauenklinik
Abteilung Gynäkologische Endokrinologie
Voßstraße 9
D-6900 Heidelberg 1

Professor Dr. phil. nat. WOLFGANG MERZ
Institut für Biochemie II
Im Neuenheimer Feld 328
D-6900 Heidelberg 1

ISBN 978-3-540-13854-9   ISBN 978-3-662-00662-7 (eBook)

DOI 10.1007/978-3-662-00662-7

2123/3130-543210

Contents

Introduction

In 1920, Hirose demonstrated the luteinising effect of placental tissue and one year later, Evans and Long described luteinised ovaries in rats treated with hypophysial extracts. In 1926, Zondek and Aschheim as well as Smith, independently of each other, showed that a gonad-stimulating hormone was secreted by the adenohypophysis. In 1927, Aschheim and Zondek found their "Prolan" in human pregnancy urine and the first reliable pregnancy test was available. In the following years it could be demonstrated that the gonadotropic hormones from pituitary and from pregnancy urin were not of identical structure. During the years 1931 - 1933 Fevold and coworkers prepared follicle stimulating hormone from sheep pituitaries which were free of other hormone activities. Already in 1934, Collip found "antihormones" in animals treated with proteinhormones from animals of another species. It could be shown that they were antibodies against these hormones and this was the future basis for the immunological era starting in 1960. The quantitative determination of gonadotropins has been performed over several decades by difficult bioassays and since 1960 immunological and later radioimmunological assays became available. Since that time a new field was opened for the studies of gonadotropins. During this time, highly purified preparations of gonadotropins were available for research and clinical treatment. I recall the first successful attempt of inducing follicle growth and ovulation by Gemzell and coworkers 1958 as well as by Lunenfeld and Bettendorf at about the same time. A further period of development started with the discovery of releasing hormones as thyreotropin releasing hormones by Guillemin's group 1969 and the gonadotropin releasing hormone (Gn - RH) also by Guillemin's group and by Schally 1972.

In order to enable the understanding of the regulatory mechanisms between the hypothalamus and the pituitary on one hand and between these central regulatory systems and the ovary, the quantitative determinations of proteo- and steroid hormones are by themselves alone not sufficient. Hypothalamic function can only be assessed indirectly, as releasing hormones cannot be measured accurately yet. A certain amount of information can be gained from functional tests with anti-estrogens and by measuring pituitary gonadotropins. The function of the pituitary, however, can be determined more easily by the measurement of its secretory products prolactin, FSH and LH as well as by the stimulatory tests TRH and Gn-RH. Nevertheless, we know only little about the close endocrine relationship of hypothalamus and pituitary. Functional disorders on this level cause most often abnormalities of the female cycle. Sometimes you can find straightforward causes such as hyperprolactinemia, hyperandrogenism or failure of an endocrine organ. In order to be able to clarify several functional disorders of the regulatory mechanism of hypothalamus and pituitary together with their effect on the gonads precise knowledge of gonadotropin action on the cell is necessary. Such studies will offer new aspects of organspecific regulation and action of hormones. Thereby it may become possible to define more accurately some disturbances of the menstrual cycle such as hypothalamic or hypophyseal dysfunction. Relating to clinics, we will have some contributions to the up-to-date state of the use of GnRH in induction of ovulation. Following some initial problems this novel method of treatment has proved to be safer, better controlled and more effective than HMG therapy. There has been a rapid development in the field of GnRH agonists and more recently also antagonists.

In the future, these substances will have their therapeutical role in hormone-dependent diseases, whereby gonadal function needs to be abolished such as in endometrial, breast and prostatic cancer. It is most likely that GnRH analogues will increasingly gain importance as a female as well as male contraceptive.

Heidelberg, October 1984   Prof. Dr. med. B.Runnebaum

Receptors and Actions of Gonadotropin Releasing Hormone (GnRH) in the Anterior Pituitary Gland

L. Kiesel[1], E. Loumaye[2], and K. J. Catt[3]

[1] Department of Obstetrics & Gynecology, Voßstr. 9, D-6900 Heidelberg
[2] Department of Obstetrics & Gynecology, University of Louvain,
   5330, Ave. Em. Mounier, 53, B-1200 Brussels
[3] Endocrinology and Reproduction Research Branch, National Institutes of Health, Building 10,
   Room 8C-404, Bethesda, MD 20205, USA

INTRODUCTION

Since the isolation of the hypothalamic decapeptide responsible for the stimulation of gonadotropic secretion by the anterior pituitary gland, many analogs of the gonadotropin-releasing hormone (GnRH) have been synthesized with the aim of providing more potent agonists and antagonists for the pharmacological regulation of gonadotropin secretion in man and experimental animals. It was soon recognized that GnRH agonists are highly effective in desensitizing the gonadotrophs and reducing their secretory capacity, following the initial stimulatory action on gonadotropin release. This effect of GnRH was first observed in animals treated with the releasing hormone (Rippel et al. 1974) and its agonist analogs, and has been extensively applied in experimental and clinical situations (De Koning et al. 1978; Belchetz et al. 1978; Corbin et al. 1978; Sandow et al. 1979). In particular, the ability of GnRH super-agonists to desensitize the pituitary gland has been used to suppress gonadotropin release in patients with disorders related to excessive or unwanted secretion of gonadotropins or gonadal steroids (Nillius et al. 1978; Labrie et al. 1978).

The analysis of GnRH receptors was initially impeded by the lack of suitable radioactive probes to label the specific receptor sites and to characterize their binding properties. Several early studies on this topic demonstrated that satisfactory radioligand binding studies could not be performed with radioiodinated or tritiated derivatives of the native hypothalamic decapeptide. However, this problem was overcome by the use of synthetic super-agonist GnRH derivatives to prepare ^{125}I-labeled ligands for the measurement and characterization of receptors for the measurement and characterization of receptors for GnRH in the anterior pituitary gland (Spona 1973; Clayton et al. 1978).

This review will survey recent studies on the properties and regulation of GnRH receptors and the mechanisms by which GnRH stimulates gonadotropin secretion.

TARGET-CELL ACTIONS OF GNRH

Following its synthesis in neurones located in the medial preoptic area of the hypothalamus, GnRH is transported by axoplasmic flow in nerve fibers which terminate in the palisade zone of the median eminence. There, the decapeptide is released in a pulsatile manner into the portal circulation and stimulates the secretion of luteinizing hormone (LH) and follicle-stimulating hormone (FSH) from the gonadotrophs of the anterior pituitary gland. Recently, GnRH peptides have been found to exert effects not only on the anterior pituitary gland but also on other tissues including the ovary and testis of certain species , and the brain and sympathetic nervous system. The gonadotrophs upon which GnRH acts via its specific receptors located in the plasma membrane can be readily identified by electron microscopy and immunocytochemical labeling of the granules which contain gonadotropins. The native decapeptide is rapidly degraded by peptidases in the hypothalamus and the pituitary gland, particularly at the 6-7 and 9-10 bonds (Koch et al. 1974; Marks and Stern 1974). Many analogs of GnRH have been prepared by substition at these two positions to provide more potent compounds which are resistant to enzymatic degradation. Among the most frequently used analogs are those with D-amino acid substituents in the 6th position (e.g., (D-Ser-(t-Bu^6) derivatives) and also at the C-terminus, by deletion of the Gly^{10} residues and termination as the N-ethylamide.

Several of these analogs, such as (D-Ala^6) and (D-Ser(t-Bu^6))des-Gly^{10}-GnRH-N-ehtylamide (GnRH-A) have been used for labeling receptors after derivation with radioactive iodine. The proliferation of synthetic peptides with activity as GnRH agonists and antagonists indicates the potential importance of these compounds for experimental and therapeutic use. The original antagonists formed by substitution at the 2 position were relatively low in potency, but more recent modifications have provided very potent antagonists which may become clinically important in the control of pituitary function.

ANALYSIS OF GNRH RECEPTORS WITH RADIOIODINATED SUPER-AGONISTS

Radioiodinated GnRH super-agonists have been useful in receptor analysis because of their high affinity and biological activity, and their relatively slow degradation in receptor assays. The use of such derivatives for the characterization of pituitary GnRH binding sites has defined a homogenous set of receptors with equilibrium affinity constant (Ka) of 4×10^9 M^{-1}. This type of labeling has also been used in competitive radioligand assays to evaluate the properties of GnRH analogs, and to compare their receptor binding affinities and biological activities (Clayton and Catt 1981a). Thus, a comparison between radioligand binding and the release of gonadotropins from cultured pituitary cells shows a good correlation between the ED$_{50}$ for biological activity and the receptor binding affinity (Kd) for a wide range of peptide agonists from GnRH (the least potent) to the (D-amino acid^6)-des-Gly^{10} -N-ethylamide peptides (the most potent). Such radioligand assays can be used to measure the physiological changes in the concentration of GnRH receptors in pituitary cells that occur during development and throughout the estrus cycle and post-partum period of lactation in the rat (Loumaye et al. 1982).

PHYSIOLOGICAL REGULATIONS OF PITUITARY GNRH RECEPTORS

In the rat pituitary gland, GnRH undergo marked changes during the estrous cycle with an increase during proestrus and a fall around the time of the LH surge. This cyclical change, in which a two-fold increase in GnRH receptors during the estrus cycle, demonstrates that substantial variations in receptor expression occur under physiological conditions (Clayton et al. 1980). GnRH receptors were also examined during lactation, when the reduced secretion of gonadotropin is believed to be due to decreased release of GnRH from the hypothalamus. In lactating rats, pituitary GnRH receptors were much lower than in normal cycling animals, as were the serum LH concentrations (Fig. 1). Thus, it appears that a reduction in the concentration of GnRH impinging on the pituitary gland leads to a decrease in both pituitary GnRH receptors and gonadotropin secretion. Such findings have led to studies on the control of GnRH receptors and the factors that could be responsible for their up-and down-regulation in various states of reproductive function.

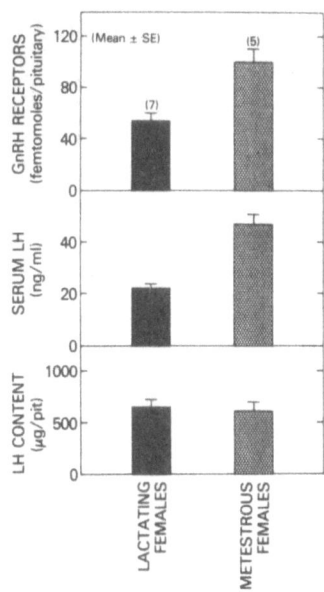

Fig. 1. Pituitary GnRH receptor content (upper panel) of glands obtained from female rats suckling 8 - 10 pups between 5 and 15 days of age (■), and metestrous females (▨). Receptor number determined as described in Fig. 8 legend. Serum LH (nanograms per ml RP-1) and pituitary LH (micrograms RP-1 per gland) are shown in the middle and lower panels, respectively. (Reproduced with permission from Clayton RN & Catt KJ (1981 a), Endocrine Reviews 2:186)

EFFECTS OF CASTRATION ON GNRH RECEPTORS

In both female and male rats, castration is followed by a 2- to 3-fold increase in GnRH receptors within a few days. This increase in receptors can be prevented by treatment with the appropriate gonadal steroid, either estrogen or androgen (Clayton and Catt 1981b). These findings suggest that any increase or decrease in GnRH secretion is accompanied by a parallel change in pituitary GnRH receptors. This process can be modulated by gonadal hormones, and in the rat pituitary gland the changes in GnRH receptors appear to be directly proportional to the concentration of the ligand in the hypothalamic-pituitary portal system. Studies designed to test this proposal have shown that pituitary GnRH receptors are directly dependent upon hypothalamic GnRH secretion in the rat. Thus, the increase in GnRH receptors after gonadectomy can be prevented by the placement of a median eminence lesion at the same time as castration. Also, treatment of the lesioned animals with small doses of GnRH caused an increase in pituitary receptors (Fig. 2). Such experiments have shown that blocking the formation or action of endogenous GnRH prevents the increase in receptors; conversely, replacement by exogenous GnRH reproduces the increase in receptors. This increase in receptors can also be abolished by administering either GnRH antagonists or antisera to block the action of the endogenous peptide, again indicating that the hypothalamic secretion of GnRH is responsible for the control of pituitary GnRH receptors (Frager et al. 1981). Such studies have indicated that the GnRH receptor can be positively modulated by the prevailing concentration of its regulatory ligand in the portal circulation.

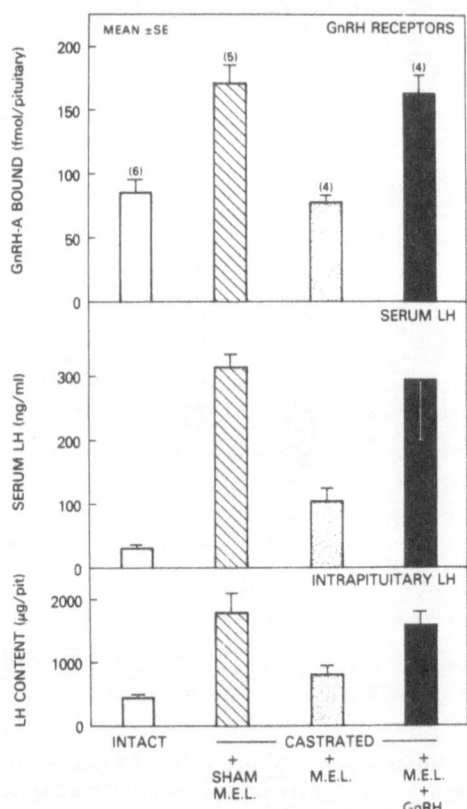

Fig. 2. Effect of destructive median eminence lesions (MEL) on pituitary GnRH receptors, serum LH, and pituitary LH responses to castration in adult male rats. One group of MEL castrated rats received thrice daily sc injections (240 ng/dose) of GnRH, beginning from the time of MEL placement. Values are the mean ± SE of data from the number of animals shown in parentheses above each bar. (Reproduced with permission from Clayton RN & Catt KJ (1981 a), Endocrine Reviews 2:186)

IN VITRO REGULATION OF GNRH RECEPTORS

To analyze the control of GnRH receptors in vitro, the effects of GnRH and its analogs upon GnRH receptors were studied during incubation with cultured rat anterior pituitary cells. In cells exposed to the peptide for 8 hours there was a consistent increase in receptors at higher concentrations of GnRH (Fig. 3). Such a biphasic and concentration-dependent effect of GnRH on its receptors may be responsible for the increase in GnRH receptors during the proestrus period of the rat cycle. It could also explain the subsequent decrease in receptors just prior to the LH surge, when there may be increased secretion of GnRH from the hypothalamus. In contrast, a GnRH antagonist with the same binding affinity as the natural GnRH decapeptide had no effect upon the receptors (Loumaye and Catt 1983). In studies on the concentration-dependence of different doses of GnRH, there was biphasic regulation of receptors by several agonist analogs. The super-agonists cause the same biphasic response, though with more pronounced effects than the native peptide. In general, the pituitary GnRH receptors can be increased by up to 70% by moderate elevations in GnRH concentration, and undergo a decrease at higher concentrations of GnRH.

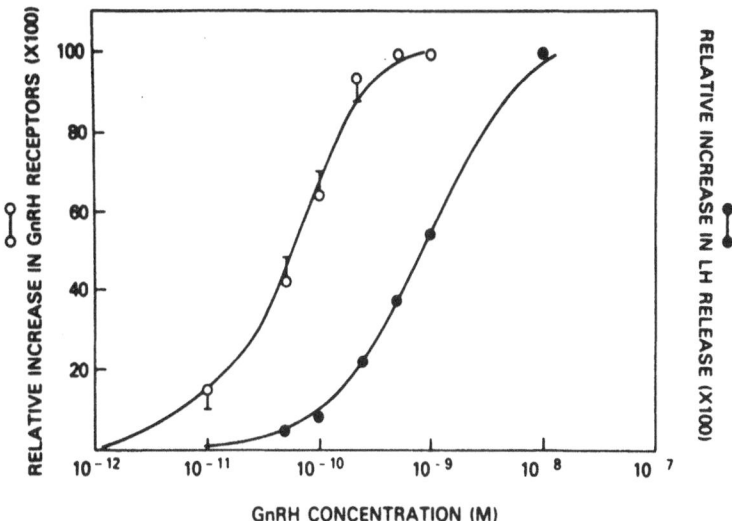

Fig. 3. Dose-response curves for GnRH-induced receptor up-regulation (o—o) and LH release (●—●). Cultured pituitary cells were incubated with several concentrations of native GnRH for 8 h, then aliquots of the culture medium were assayed from LH content and cells were assayed for GnRH receptor content. The dose-response curves are the combined results of five experiments. The ED_{50} values obtained by the ALLFIT program for GnRH up regulation and LH release were $7.4 \pm 1.5 \times 10^{-11}$ M and $9.9 \pm 0.7 \times 10^{-10}$ M, respectively. (Reproduced with permission from Loumaye E & Catt KJ (1983) J Biol Chem 258:12002)

TIME COURSE OF GNRH ACTION UPON RECEPTORS

The kinetics of the effects of GnRH upon its receptors were analyzed for up to 10 h in cultured pituitary cells during exposure to GnRH or a weak antagonist derivative. After addition of GnRH, the increase in receptors measured at 6 to 8 h was found to be preceded by an acute decrease in receptors. This early loss of sites was followed by a return to the control level and then by an increase in receptors. Thus, GnRH receptors undergo a complicated cycle after occupancy by the agonist ligand, with an initial phase of depletion followed by regeneration or return to normal and a subsequent increase in receptor number. In contrast, the GnRH antagonist had no effect on either GnRH receptors or basal LH secretion (Fig. 4). The stimulation of LH secretion by GnRH occurred mainly during the first 1 to 3 h and thus corresponded more to the stage of down-regulation rather than to the later phase of receptor replenishment and up regulation.

A comparison was made between the actions of GnRH upon down- and up-regulation of receptors, and the effect of a secretory stimulus which does not involve receptor activation. In cells exposed to high concentrations of K^+ to cause membrane depolarization, release of LH was followed by receptor up regulation with no preceding loss of receptors. This finding suggests that the loss of receptors during the phase of down-regulation is mediated by the occupancy of receptor sites by the stimulatory ligand. Thus, if there is occupancy of receptor sites by the stimulatory ligand by an antagonist which does not activate the target cell, or if a non-receptor stimulus such as K^+ is used, the initial phase of receptor loss or down regulation is not observed.

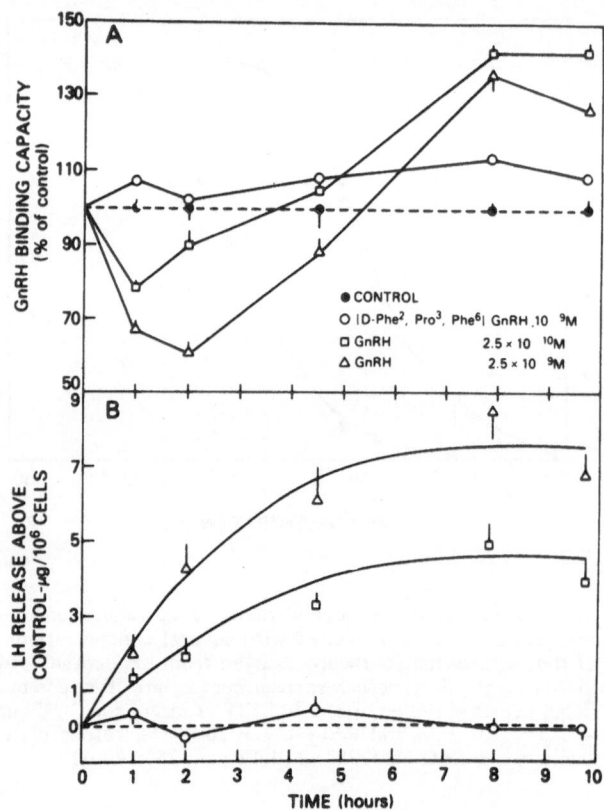

<u>Fig. 4.</u> Kinetics of receptor regulation in cells incubated with GnRH and a GnRH antagonist. Cultured pituitary cells were treated with native GnRH ($\square$,$\blacktriangle$) or with the D-Phe[2], Pro[3], Phe[6]-labeled antagonist (O). At selected times, an aliquot of the culture medium was removed for assay of LH concentration, and the cells were assayed for GnRH binding capacity. <u>A</u>, GnRH binding capacity expressed as a percentage of the control value in nontreated cells. <u>B</u>, LH release expressed in $\mu g/10^6$ cells above the release by control cells. (Reproduced with permission from Loumaye E & Catt KJ (1983) J Biol Chem 258:12002)

ROLE OF PROTEIN SYNTHESIS IN RECEPTOR UP-REGULATION

Pituitary cells were exposed to GnRH in the presence and absence of cycloheximide or actinomycin D (Loumaye and Catt 1983). The action of GnRH was typical: an initial decrease in receptors was followed by a return to normal, and then by a delayed increase in receptors. In the presence of cycloheximide there was still the early decrease in receptors and the accompanying release of LH, but there was no subsequent increase in receptors. However, when the cells were washed to remove the cycloheximide there was a delayed increase in receptors at about the same rate as in cells treated with GnRH alone, but with a delay of several hours. These observations indicated that the return of receptors is dependent on protein synthesis, but whether this required for the restoration of receptors themselves or for some other protein involved in the replenishment process is not yet known.

KINETICS OF HORMONE ACTION IN PERIFUSED PITUITARY CELLS

When increasing concentrations of GnRH are applied to pituitary cells suspended in a gel column, there is a progressive increase in LH release. In this system, a dose-response curve is obtained with GnRH concentrations up to 100 nM, from concentrations as low as 10 pM. If GnRH pulses are repeated for many hours, the cells continue to respond with pulsatile release of LH into the perifusion medium (Knobil et al. 1980).When compared to the action of native GnRH, super-agonists such as (D-Ala^6)GnRH-EA and (D-Ser(t-Bu^6)) GnRH-EA cause a similar initial peak in LH release, but the duration of the LH response is more protracted. The more extensive secretion of LH is attributable to higher binding affinity of the super-agonists for the GnRH receptors, with correspondingly slower dissociation leading to a more prolonged action upon gonadotropin release.

If GnRH agonists are applied for a prolonged time, the initial peak of LH release is followed by a fall despite the continued exposure to the agonist. Thereafter the cells are relatively refractory to further stimulation by the same peptide. This phenomenon has been observed in several in vitro studies and reflects GnRH induced desensitization of the pituitary cells. Since other stimuli such as high K$^+$ or calcium ionophores will still elicit LH release, this appears to be a specific, receptor-mediated effect of GnRH and its agonists.

The in vivo counterpart of this phenomenon was observed by Knobil et al. (1980) in Rhesus monkeys, when attempting to maintain gonadotropin secretion in animals with hypothalamic lesions. Whereas continuous infusions of GnRH were not effective in this regard, intermittent treatment with pulses of GnRH every 1 to 2 hours successfully maintained gonadotropin secretion. Subsequently, many studies in animals and man have shown that pulsatile presentation of GnRH to the pituitary cells is essential for the stimulation of a sustained gonadotropin response.

TURNOVER AND FATE OF THE GNRH RECEPTORS

The fate of the GnRH receptors has been studied by several techniques, including the use of fluorescent GnRH derivatives such as rhodamine-labeled (D-Lys^6)GnRH (Pelletier et al. 1982). In cultured rat pituitary cells, only a small proportion of the cells took up this fluorescent ligand, since only 10% of the cells in the pituitary gland are gonadotrophs. After 10 to 20 minutes there was an increasing clustering and clumping of this material, giving the impression that the bound ligand reorganized in a way that leads to uptake into the cell. This question has been resolved by electron microscopy (EM) to analyze the fate of ^{125}I-labeled GnRH agonist which has been injected into the intact rat and taken up by the pituitary. EM pictures of the grain distribution in pituitary cells has shown that the labeled agonist is densely concentrated in about 10% of the pituitary cells, and there are very few grains in the other pituitary cells. The labeled agonist binds specifically to gonadotrophs, and it is evident that some of the grains are on the plasma membrane while others are inside the cells and sometimes associated with secretory granules and other organelles.

Similar studies by Pelletier et al. (1982) showed that the radioactive hormone is rapidly internalized, and that many of the grains are inside the cell within 10 to 15 minutes. Similarly, Naor et al. (1981) found at 30 min. that almost 75% of the hormone was inside the cell, associated with various organelles including lysosomes, Golgi apparatus and secretory granules. The association with granules has led to the speculation that secretory granules might be involved in the receptor recycling process. This phenomenon was further suspected because sometimes the secretory granules appear to contain binding sites for GnRH. However, our studies in cultured cells do not support the idea that granules are a source of receptors during replenishment, since hormone secretion occurs quite rapidly while receptors do not increase until many hours later. For this and other reasons it is unlikely that secretory granules are involved in receptor turn-over in the pituitary gonadotrophs. It appears likely that internalization in gonadotrophs occurs in a similar manner to that observed in many other ligand stimulated cells. Thus, the ligand becomes associated with the receptor and is then taken up through a coated-pit mechanism or other means, and after endocytosis can go through two possible pathways, either degradation or recycling to the plasma membrane.

It is well known that many molecules that are important for transport (e.g. LDL and transferrin receptors) are continuously recycled. On the other hand, most of the peptide hormone receptors are thought to undergo degradation, although some recycling may occur. Such degradation of sites is probably responsible for much of the down-regulation of receptors that occurs in hormone-responsive tissues. The ability of GnRH to desensitize the pituitary cells probably depends in part on changes in receptor number and to a greater degree on receptor-mediated desensitization. The inhibition of gonadotropin release by GnRH agonists has been shown to influence several aspects of reproduction (Nillius et al. 1978; Das & Talwar 1983) and puberty (Comite et al. 1981; Furr and Nicholson 1982). Various steroid-dependent disorders, including tumors of the mammary gland, prostate cancer (Tolis et al. 1982; Santen et al. 1984), and endometriosis (Lemay and Quesnel 1982), have been ameliorated by suppression of the pituitary gland with GnRH agonists. The other major use of GnRH as a gonadotropin suppressant is in the control of fertility. This area is still under development, but the daily intra-nasal administration of a super-agonist analog has been quite effective in preventing ovulation in normal women. Although a major application of GnRH agonists has been for their suppressive effect on pituitary-gonadal function, there will probably be an increased use of antagonists for this purpose in the future. However, the extent to which the suppressive effect of agonist desensitization can be improved upon has yet to be determined.

MECHANISM OF ACTION OF GNRH

Peptide hormones and transmitters are often classified according to their mechanisms of action. Thus, the cAMP-dependent hormones, the calcium and cGMP related hormones, and the modulator dependent hormones can be distinguished by the membrane-associated response that mediate their cellular actions (Berridge 1981). GnRH appears to belong to the family of Ca-dependent ligands whose actions require calcium and often involve increased formation of cGMP, and are also associated with and increased turnover of phospholipids. However, despite the fact that GnRH does increase cGMP levels, this cyclic nucleotide does not appear to be an intermediate in the action of GnRH on the release of LH. If the increase in level of cGMP is blocked by compounds such as mycophenolic acid, there is no impairment of LH release (Naor et al. 1980a). Thus, cGMP appears to be a concomitant of the activation of the gonadotroph rather than a part of the mechanism of LH secretion. The effect of GnRH on LH release is highly calcium-dependent, and GnRH has very little effect on either LH or cGMP in the absence of extracellular Ca^{++}. However, with increasing concentrations of medium calcium there is an increased response to GnRH in cultured pituitary cells (Naor et al. 1980).

ROLE OF ARACHIDONIC ACID IN THE MECHANISM OF ACTION OF GNRH

We have previously observed that release of arachidonic acid, possibly via activation of phospholipase A_2, occurs when pituitary cells are stimulated by GnRH. Thus, cells pre-labeled with ^{3}H-arachidonic acid and incubated with GnRH show a progressive release of arachidonic acid with time. The release of arachidonic acid from cells stimulated with GnRH occurs rapidly, and is associated with LH release. This suggests that GnRH stimulated phospholipid degradation and turnover, and release of arachidonic acid and its products could be important components of the LH release mechanism. Earlier studies by Naor et al. (1981) showed that the prostaglandin branch of the arachidonate metabolic pathway does not appear to be involved in the actions of GnRH upon pituitary gonadotrophs. However, more recent evidence has indicated that the other major pathway of arachidonic acid metabolism, leading to lipoxygenase products such as hydroxy fatty acids (HETEs) and their leukotriene derivatives, is more important in the actions of GnRH (Kiesel and Catt 1984a; Farese 1984).

When the release of LH was measured after the addition of GnRH or arachidonic acid, the fatty acid mimicked the effect of GnRH and was not an additive stimulus upon LH release. Addition of indomethacin, which itself has little effect on LH release, did not block the actions of arachidonic acid or GnRH (Fig. 5). Thus, it appears that arachidonic acid or its metabolites are

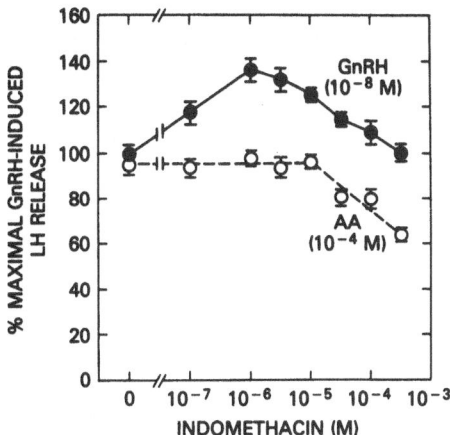

Fig. 5. Addition of indomethacin (10^{-7} - 3 x 10^{-4} M) to gonadotrophs stimulated by GnRH (10^{-8} M) or arachidonic acid (AA, 10^{-4} M).

involved in the release of LH, but that such metabolites are not products of the cyclooxygenase pathway. To evaluate the involvement of the lipoxygenase pathway in GnRH action, studies were performed with putative inhibitors of the lipoxygenase pathway. The effect of GnRH on LH release could be blocked by lipoxygenase inhibitors including NDGA and ETYA, whereas indomethacin has little effect or causes some stimulation of LH release in GnRH treated cells. This provides indirect evidence that the lipoxygenase pathway may be involved in the mechanism of action of GnRH, but which component of the pathway is involved is not yet known.

Examination of the effects of several 5-lipoxygenase products and leukotrienes revealed that most of these agents do not mimic the effect of GnRH on LH release. The one compound other than arachidonic acid that does have an effect on LH release is 5-HETE (Kiesel and Catt 1984a; Farese 1984). Whereas arachidonic acid consistently causes LH release, other hydroxy fatty acids including 11-HETE, 12-HETE and 15-HETE had no effect on LH release. However, 5-HETE partially reproduced the action of arachidonic acid (Fig. 6) and could be involved in the mechanism of LH release.

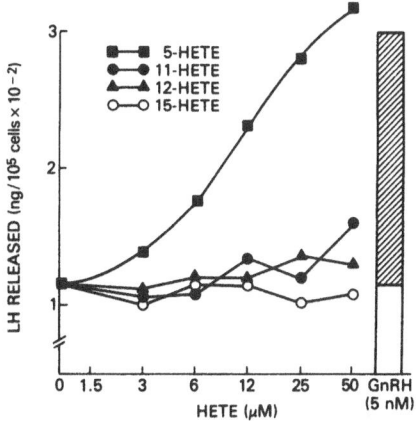

Fig. 6. Effect of different HETE metabolites on LH release. Cultured pituitary cells were incubated with various concentrations of the substance indicated or with 5nM of GnRH for 3 hr, and LH released into the medium was determined by radioimmunoassay.

12

The effect of arachidonic acid on LH release was not accompanied by a corresponding increase in cGMP production (Kiesel & Catt 1984a). This contrasts with the combined cGMP and LH responses to GnRH, and suggests that arachidonic acid acts at a site later than the point at which cGMP is regulated.

ROLE OF PHOSPHOLIPIDS IN GNRH ACTION

Several phospholipids can give rise to arachidonic acid which may act either directly or via a lipoxygenase metabolite upon granule fusion to promote LH release. Although the exact nature of this mechanism is still unknown, it is now widely accepted that phosphatidylinositol turnover through the phosphatidylinositol- diacyglycerol-phosphatidic acid (PI-DG-PA) cycle is often associated with Ca^{++} mobilization within cells in which elevated cytosolic Ca^{++} leads to responses such as exocytosis (Lapetina et al. 1981). In recent studies (Kiesel and Catt 1984b) on the role of PI-DG-PA cycle products on LH release, we observed that PA can reproduce the actions of GnRH upon both LH release and cGMP production (Fig. 7).

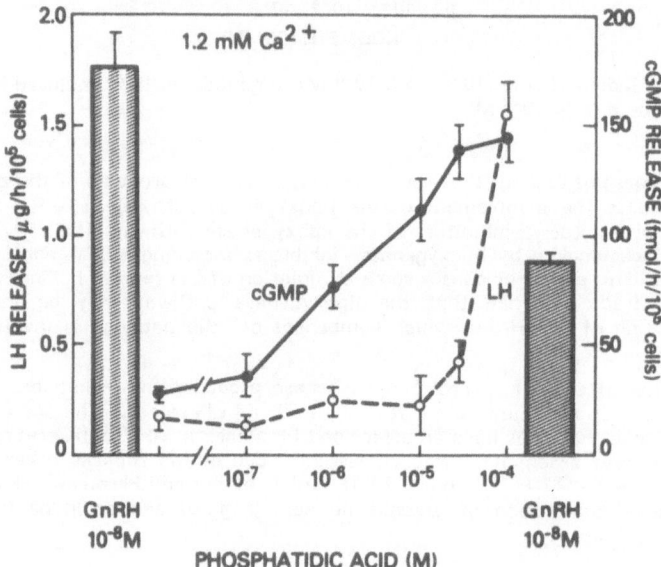

Fig. 7. Stimulation of LH release and cGMP production by phosphatidic acid. Cultured gonadotrophs (3×10^4 cells/well) were incubated in Medium 199 (1.2 mM Ca^{2+}) containing 25 mM Hepes and 0.2 mM 3-isobutyl-1-methylxanthine in the presence of phosphatidic acid (10^{-7} to 10^{-4} M). After 2 h, the supernatants were removed and LH and cGMP were determined by radioimmunoassay.

Furthermore, in pituitary cells labeled with radioactive ^{32}Phosphorus and treated with GnRH, there was an increased rate of incorporation into phosphatidylinositol (PI) and phosphatidic acid (PA), but no increase in the labeling of phosphtidylcholine (Fig. 8).

These findings suggest that GnRH is causing increased turnover of the PI-DG-PA cycle, in which PI is degraded by phospholipase C with cleavage of the inositol moiety and formation of diacyglycerol (DG) and subsequently PA which is resynthesized to PI. This could operate in the gonadotroph, as recently suggested for the platelet by Lapetina et al. (1981), to promote arachidonate metabolism by the following mechanism. The primary hormonal stimulus may activate receptors to cause phospholipase C-dependent cleavage of PI into DG and subsequently PA. The PA formed could act as a calcium ionophore to increase the activity of phospholipase A_2, which acts on various phospholipids to cleave off arachidonic acid, which would then be converted to its active metabolites. Several of these steps are known to occur in the pituitary cell during stimulation by GnRH, and this sequence of events may constitute the mechanism by which GnRH act upon its target cells to elicit gonadotropin secretion. The extent to which this

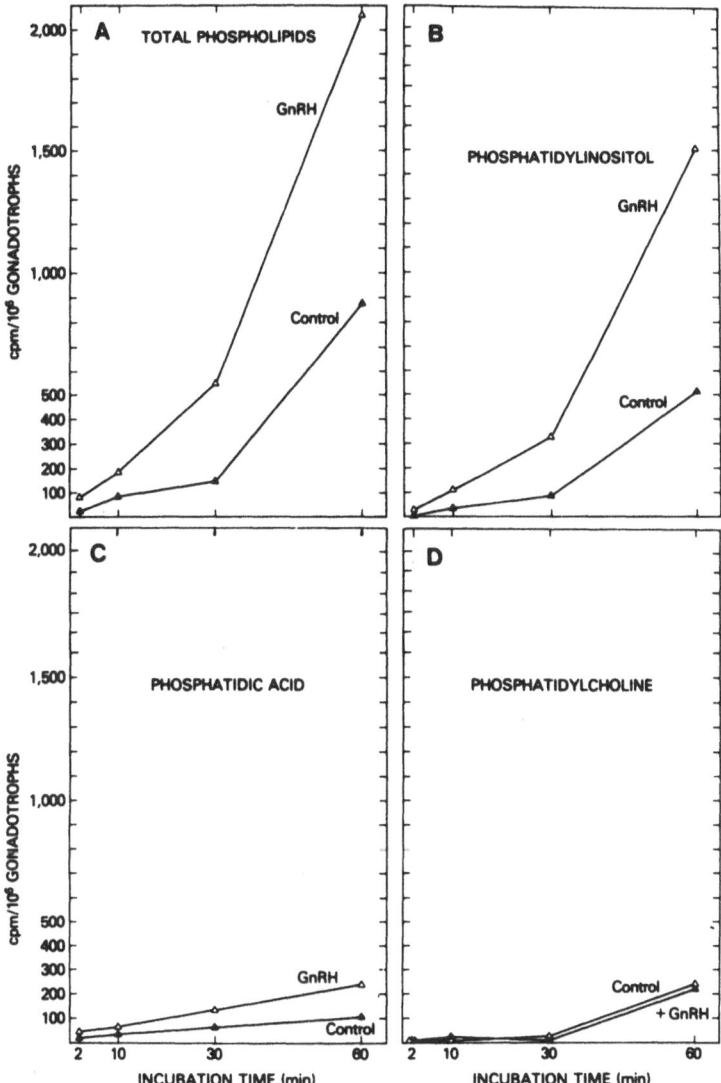

Fig. 8. Incorporation of $^{32}P_i$ into phospholipids of purified gonadotrophs (A) total phospholipids; (B) phosphatidylinositol; (C) phosphatidic acid; and (D) phosphatidylcholine. Following the addition of 50 µCi $^{32}P_i$ to 2-day cultured gonadotrophs (5 x 10^5 cells/well), GnRH was added and incubations were continued for up to 60 min in Medium 199 containing 25 mM Hepes and without inorganic phosphate. Radiolabeled phospholipids were extracted and separated.

mechanism and that related to the formation of arachidonic acid metabolites jointly participate in the processes of granule exocytosis and hormone secretion is currently under active investigation and will be more clearly defined in the near future.

ACKNOWLEDGEMENTS

The investigations were partially supported by the Deutsche Forschungsgemeinschaft, Bonn-Bad Godesberg, as a DFG grant to Dr. L. Kiesel. We wish to thank Mrs. J. LaRocca and M. Neidig for typing the manuscript. The technical assistance of Mr. A. Baukal is gratefully acknowledged.

REFERENCES

Belchetz PE, Plant TM, Nakai Y, Keogh EJ, Knobil E (1978) Hypophysial responses to continuous and intermittent delivery of hypothalamic gonadotropin releasing hormone. Science 202:631

Berridge MJ (1981) Phosphatidylinositol hydrolysis: a multifunctional transducing mechanism. Mol Cell Endocrinol 24:115

Clayton RN, Shakespear RA, Marshall JC (1978) LHRH binding to purified pituitary plasma membranes: absence of adenylate cyclase activation. Mol Cell Endocrinol 11:63

Clayton RN, Solano AR, Garcia-Vela A, Dufau ML, Catt KJ (1980) Regulation of pituitary receptors for gonadotropin-releasing hormone during the rat estrous cycle. Endocrinology 107:699

Clayton RN, Catt KJ (1981a) Gonadotropin-releasing hormone receptors: characterization, physiological regulation, and relationship to reproductive function. Endocrine Reviews 2:186

Clayton RN, Catt KJ (1981b) Regulation of pituitary gonadotropin-releasing hormone receptors by gonadal hormones. Endocrinology 108:887

Comite F, Cutler GB, Rivier J, Vale WW, Loriaux DL, Crowley WF (1981) Short-term treatment of idiopathic precocious puberty with a long-acting analogue of luteinizing hormone-releasing hormone. N Engl J Med 305:1546

Corbin A, Beattie CW, Tracy J, Jones R, Foell TJ, Yardley J, Rees RWA (1978) The anti-reproductive pharmacology of LHRH and agonistic analogues. Int Fertil 12:81

Das C, Talwar GP (1983) Pregnancy-terminating action of a luteinizing hormone-releasing agonist D-Ser(Bu^t)^{6}desGly^{10}ProEA in baboons. Fertil Steril 39:218

De Koning J, van Dieten JAMJ, van Rees GP (1978) Refractoriness of the pituitary gland after continuous exposure to luteinizing hormone-releasing hormone. J Endocrinol 79:311

Farese RV (1984) Phospholipids as intermediates in hormonal action. Mol Cell Endocrinol 35:1

Frager MS, Pieper DR, Tonetta S, Duncan JA, Marshall JC (1981) Pituitary gonadotropin-releasing hormone (GnRH) receptors: effects of castration, steroid replacement, and the role of GnRH in modulating receptors in the rat. J Clin Invest 67:615

Furr BJA, Nicholson RI (1982) Use of analogues of luteinizing hormone-releasing hormone for treatment of cancer. J Reprod Fertil 64:529

Kiesel L, Catt KJ (1984a) Stimulation of luteinizing hormone release and cyclic nucleotide production by arachidonic acid in cultured pituitary gonadotrophs (submitted for publication)

Kiesel L, Catt KJ (1984b) Phosphatidic acid and the calcium-dependent actions of gonadotropin-releasing hormone in pituitary gonadotrophs. Arch Biochem Biophys 231:202

Knobil E, Plant TM, Wildt L, Belchetz PE, Marshall G (1980) Control of the rhesus monkey menstrual cycle: permissive role of hypothalamic gonadotropin-releasing hormone. Science 207:1371

Koch Y, Baram T, Chobsieng P, Fridkin M (1974) Enzymatic degradation of LHRH by hypothalamic tissue. Biochem Biophys Res Com 61:95

Labrie F, Auclair C, Cusan L, Kelly PA, Pelletier G, Ferland L (1978) Inhibitory effect of LHRH and its agonists on testicular gonadotropin receptors and spermatogenesis in the rat. Int J Androl (Suppl 2) 1:303

Lapetina EG, Billah NM, Cuatrecasas P (1981) The phosphatidylinositol cycle and the regulation of arachidonic acid production. Nature 292:367

Lemay A, Quesnel G (1982) Potential new treatment of endometriosis: reversible inhibition of pituitary-ovarian function by chronic intranasal administration of a luteinizing hormone-releasing hormone (LHRH) agonist. Fertil Steril 38:376

Loumaye E, Naor Z, Catt KJ (1982) Binding affinity and biological activity of gonadotropin-releasing hormone agonists in isolated pituitary cells. Endocrinology 111:730

Loumaye E, Catt KJ (1983) Agonist-induced regulation of pituitary receptors for gonadotropin-releasing hormone. J Biol Chem 258:12002

Marks N, Stern F (1974) Enzymatic mechanisms for the inactivation of LHRH. Biochem Biophys Res Comm 61:1458

Naor Z, Catt KJ (1980) Independent actions of gonadotropin releasing hormone upon cyclic GMP production and luteinizing hormone release. J Biol Chem 255:342

Naor Z, Leifer AM, Catt KJ (1980) Calcium-dependent actions of gonadotropin-releasing hormone on pituitary guanosine 3',5'-monophosphate production and gonadotropin release. Endocrinology 107:1438

Naor Z, Atlas D, Clayton RN, Forman DS, Amsterdam A, Catt KJ (1981) Fluorescent derivative of gonadotropin-releasing hormone: visualization of hormone-receptor interaction in cultured pituitary cells. J Biol Chem 256:3049

Naor Z, Catt KJ (1981) Mechanism of action of gonadotropin-releasing hormone. J Biol Chem 256:2226

Naor Z, Vanderhoek JY, Lindner HR, Catt KJ (1983) Arachidonic acid products as possible mediators of the action of gonadotropin-releasing hormone. In: Samuelson B, Paoletti R, Ramwell P (eds) Advances in Prostaglandin, Thromboxane and Leukotriene Research 12:259

Nillius SJ, Bergquist C, Wide L (1978) Inhibition of ovulation in women by chronic treatment with a stimulatory LRH analogue, a new approach to birth control. Contraception 17:537

Pelletier G, Dubé D, Guy J, Séguin C, Lefèbre FA (1982) Binding and internalization of a luteinizing hormone-releasing hormone agonist by rat gonadotrophic cells. A radioautographic study. Endocrinology 111:1068

Rippel RH, Johnson ES, White WF (1974) Effect of consecutive injections of synthetic gonadotropin-releasing hormone on LH release in anestrous and ovariectomized ewes. J Anim Sci 39:907

Sandow J, van Rechenberg W, Kuhl H, Baumann R, Krauss B, Jerzabek G, Kille S (1979) Inhibitory control of the pituitary LH secretion by LHRH in male rats. Horm Res 11:303

Santen RJ, Demers LM, Max DT, Smith J, Stein BS, Glode LM (1984) Long term effects of administration of a gonadotropin releasing hormone superagonist in men with prostatic carcinoma. J Clin Endocr Metabol 58:397

Spona J (1973) LHRH interaction with pituitary plasma membrane. FEBS Lett 34:24

Tolis G, Achman D, Stellos A, Mehta A, Labrie F, Fazekas ATA, Comarn-Schally AV (1982) Tumor growth inhibition in patients with prostatic carcinoma treated with luteinizing hormone-releasing hormone agonists. Proc Natl Acad Sci USA 79:1658

Perpetual Feedback Effect in the Neurons of the Arcuate Nucleus Due to Gonadal Atrophy

G. Ule and K. Schwechheimer

Institut für Neuropathologie der Universität, Im Neuenheimer Feld 220-221, D-6900 Heidelberg

In a case of infantile hemochromatosis accompanied with hypogonadotropic hypogonadism, ULE and WALTER observed peculiar phenomenons restricted to the nuclei of the arcuate nucleus neurons. Theses comprise nucleolar augmentation, duplication and vacuolation and intranuclear cytoplasm invaginations. They were interpreted as a perpetual feedback effect due to gonadal atrophy with loss of Leydig cells. In order to elucidate this interpretation, we examined the gonads and serial sections of the unmyelinated hypothalamus by light microscopy. The series included 15 cases of women from 3o to 111 years and 7 cases of men from 29 to 82 years (Ule 1983, Ule and Schwechheimer 1983, Ule et al 1983). A remarkable coincidence between the gonadal atrophy and the increased and numerous occurence of these nuclear alterations in the arcuate nucleus was observed. Only occasionally, these findings were also singularly found in fertile women. They were more frequent in women than in men of the same age. The discrepancy is probably caused by the different involution of the ovaries and the testes. Nuclear alterations were also numerous in a women of 111 years. In this respect, the proverbal "eternal youth" of the pituitary corresponds to a comparable juvenile reagibility of the arcuate nucleus neurons which were involved in the aforementioned feedback effect. ULE and MATTFELDT recently observed this phenomenon in a case of Klinefelter's syndrome. The nuclear alterations, however, were not as abundant as in gonadal atrophy with loss of the Leydig cells. It becomes clear that also in Klinefelter's syndrome with nodular hyperplasia of the insufficient Leydig cells and a diffuse hyperplasia of the basophils, the increased production of gonadotropins is regulated by the hypothalamus.

The coincidence of gonadal atrophy and hypothalamic findings was only exceptionally missing. So the feedback effect in an alcoholic with testicular atrophy was obvious in despite of the well preserved Leydig cells. This phenomenon is best explained by the conversion of testosterone to estrogen and the increase of testosterone binding globulin. A direct toxic effect of acetoaldehyde on Leydig cells might be alternatively discussed. The feedback effect was missed in the case of 39 years old woman after ovariectomy because fo breast cancer three years prior to death. Diencephalic metastases required irradiation which caused calcified necroses in the hypothalamus as verified by autopsy.

Apart from these few exceptions the hypothalamic feedback effect due to gonadal atrophy might be expected as a rule. Electron-microscopically it was identified as intranuclear cytoplasm protrusions and immuno-cytologically it was found in arcuate neurons with and without LH-RH-like immuno-reactivity (Ule et al 1984).

REFERENCES

Ule G (1983) Morphologische Veränderungen im markarmen Hypothalamus
während der Involution und im Senium in Abhängigkeit von der Rück-
bildung der Keimdrüsen. Z Gerontol 16 : 174-176

Ule G, Mattfeldt T (1983) Zur Frage des Feedback-Effektes im Hypothalamus bei klinisch nicht erkanntem Klinefelter-Syndrom mit
iatrogenem Cushing-Syndrom. Akt Endokrinol Stoffwechsel 4 :155-159

Ule G, Schwechheimer K (1983) Morphological feedback phenomenon in
the nucleus arcuatus (infundibularis) due to gonadal atrophy. Pro-
ceedings of the 1st International Meeting on Interdisciplinary
Neuroendocrinology, Graz, June 16th-18th

Ule G, Schwechheimer K, Tschahargane C (1983) Morphological feedback-
effect on neurons of the nucl. arcuatus (sive infundibularis) and
nucl. subventricularis hypothalami due to gonadal atrophy.
Virchows Arch (Pathol Anat) 4oo : 297 - 3o8

Ule G, Schwechheimer K, Bauer M (1984) On the ultrastructure and
immunocytology of arcuate neurons with perpetuated feedback effect.
Clin Neuropathol : in press

Ule G, Walter C (1983) Morphological feedback effect on the nucleoli
of the neurons in the nucleus arcuatus (infundibularis) to hypophyseal hypogonadism in juvenile hemochromatosis. Acta Neuropathol
(Berl) 61 : 81 - 84

Contraceptive Action of LHRH and Analogues in Animals and in Humans

J. Sandow, K. Engelbart, and W. von Rechenberg

Hoechst AG, Pharmacology H 821, D-6230 Frankfurt 80

INTRODUCTION

Clinical experience with agonist analogues of luteinizing hormone-
releasing hormone (LHRH) has confirmed, that peptide contraception
may be a new readily reversible method for the control of fertility
based on regulation of events in normal reproduction. Elucidation
of the structure of LHRH in 1971 by the group of Schally provided
the initial incentive for investigation of hypothalamic-pituitary-
gonadal interaction. Structural analogues of LHRH have been developed with the intention to stimulate gonadotrophin release for prolonged time periods (agonists), or inhibit gonadadotrophin secretion by blocking the action of endogenous and exogenous LHRH (antagonists). Research on the reproductive effects of the agonists has
surprisingly revealed, that these peptides are effective and reversible contraceptives when given at supraphysiological daily doses.
The mechanisms of this contraceptive action are complex, because of
simultaneous changes in pituitary sensitivity and gonadal responsiveness to gonadotrophins (Sandow 1982a). The dose range for contraceptive action is 10-100fold higher than the minimal effective dose
stimulating LH release. The initial concept of stimulating fertility by LHRH and agonists, and inhibiting fertility by LHRH antagonists has undergone considerable change (Schally et al. 1981),
because of new physiological knowledge about the requirement for
pulsatile LHRH stimulation of the pituitary gland (Knobil 1980).
It is now accepted, that the antifertility effects observed at higher doses are an inherent property of potent agonists, but that
they are also observed after equivalent supraphysiological doses of
LHRH (Corbin and Bex 1980). Our present knowledge of the pharmacological, biochemical and clinical effects of agonists (see reviews
by Yen 1983; Sandow 1983) is sufficient to define their contraceptive potential and its limitations. For the antagonists, there is
clearly a different range of applications, and more information
about their biological tolerance and reversibility of long-term
suppression of gonadal function is urgently required to define the
contraceptive potential. An acceptable method for using a peptide
contraception will require effectiveness, reliability, reversibility and ease of administration.

INHIBITION OF SEXUAL MATURATION

In prepubertal rats, the contraceptive potential of LHRH and agonists is outlined by the marked inhibition of maturational changes.
In female rats, oestrogen secretion is reduced as shown by delayed
vaginal opening and reduced uterine weight. In male rats, weight
gain of androgen dependent organs (prostate, seminal vesicles, leva-
tor ani muscle) is inhibited, and testis weight remains lower than

in controls. During daily high dose injections of buserelin
(5 μg/rat s.c. for 8-16 weeks), male rats remain infertile, and
female rats are unable to conceive despite a normal body weight
development. When agonist treatment is stopped, the pubertal development is completed within an adequate time period, and both male
and female rats become fertile.

In juvenile male and female rats, fertility is blocked but gonadal
function is not completely suppressed by agonists. This is in contrast with the complete inhibition of idiopathic precocious puberty
in children (Comite et al. 1981). In male rats, there is a gradual
increase of the androgen dependent organs. In female rats, ovulation is not blocked, but occurs at a time when follicles are not
fully matured. The ovaries of such rats show an increased incidence
of corpora lutea, but fewer tertiary follicles. The ovarian reserve
of follicles is apparently not exhausted by the increased rate of
inappropriate ovulation. After 16 weeks of daily injections, and 8
weeks of recovery after treatment, there is a normal rate of pregnancy, and a normal litter size.

STUDIES IN ADULT RATS

The rat has been extensively studied as a test animal for antireproductive effects of LHRH agonists. As in other animal species, a
large proportion of the information is applicable to the planning
of contraceptive studies in the human, but there are significant
species differences restricting extrapolation of the findings. The
LH and FSH response to injections of LHRH and agonists is well correlated with the human response after suitable adjustment of the
effective dose for body weight, and the initial decrease of gonadotrophin secretion after repeated agonist injections (pituitary desensitization) is similar to the situation observed in men and women. However, rats differ significantly from primates in their requirement for an oestrogen priming of the pituitary before ovulation. In the rat, injection of an LHRH antiserum (passive immuni-
zation) readily blocks ovulation, whereas in primates an LHRH antiserum becomes ineffective after the preovulatory rise of oestradiol (Fraser et al. 1982). Inhibition of ovulation by LHRH antagonists is a reliable parameter of their antireproductive activity.
In contrast, it is difficult to block ovulation in rats by agonists, a high dose injection can induce ovulation from immature
follicles at any time of the oestrus cycle, and even on any day of
pregnancy. The luteolytic potential of LHRH and agonists cannot be
evaluated in normal female rats because of an extremely short luteal phase of 2 days. The physiological luteal insufficiency in rats
may be overcome by inducing pseudopregnancy by gonadotrophin injections or cervical stimulation. In the test model of the pseudopreg-
nant rat, agonists were potent luteolytic agents when given at more
than 100 times the minimal effective dose (Sandow et al. 1981a). A
luteolytic effect in the rat and rabbit is generally expressed by
termination of pregnancy, because in both species ovariectomy usually leads to abortion.

In male rats, suppression of testosterone secretion is rapidly a-
chieved by daily agonist injections (Cusan et al. 1979). The effects on spermatogenesis and fertility are variable and inconsis-
tent, because of a particular change in androgen biosynthesis observed in agonist-suppressed rats. Despite low intratesticular testosterone levels, the rate of transformation of testosterone to 5al-

pha-dihydrotestosterone (DHT) is enhanced. Male rats thus escape
from the effects of agonist suppression by activating their 5alpha-
reductase system (Bélanger et al. 1980).

STUDIES IN RABBITS AND GUINEA PIGS

In male rabbits, there is a marked response to agonist suppression,
both by injection, and by infusion from osmotic minipumps for 8
weeks. The weight of androgen-dependent organs decreases markedly,
and testes size is reduced dose-dependently. In contrast to the
male rat, where intratesticular testosterone content is lowered
to about 10% of controls, the rabbit responds only with a slight
reduction in testosterone content, despite a marked decrease in
serum testosterone. It is therefore not surprising that spermatogenesis in the rabbit is only inhibited to a limited extent.

In female rabbits, agonists have a marked dose-dependent pregnancy
terminating effect, because luteinization of all maturing follicles
deprives the pregnant rabbit of oestradiol, a luteotrophic steroid
in this species. In addition, luteolysis is enhanced by down-regulation of LH receptors in the rabbit ovary. As a reflex ovulator, the
rabbit is of limited value for antiovulatory studies, but LHRH
antagonists have been shown to prevent LH release and ovulation in
female rabbits.

The guinea pig is particularly suitable for studies on inhibition
of ovulation and luteolysis, because of its regular oestrous cycle
with a prolonged luteal phase. Treatment with buserelin 1 ug/kg
s.c. per day inhibited ovulation in adult guinea pigs and prevented
the luteal progesterone increase during two subsequent treatment
cycles. Adult female guinea pigs exposed to fertile males for 90
days were protected from pregnancy by daily injections of 4-
16 ug/kg buserelin s.c. During this treatment, the animals were
in good health and no adverse effects were observed. It is however
not possible to terminate pregnancy in guinea pigs with LHRH agonists (Puri & Csapo 1981). Surprisingly enough, adult male guinea
pigs appear to be resistant to agonist suppression even at high
doses. Whereas the acute response to an injection of 10 ug buserelin in terms of LH release and an increase in testosterone is very
marked, prolonged treatment does not reduce androgen secretion.
Daily s.c. injections of 10-100 ug/kg for 12 weeks or continuous
infusion of 20 ug/kg/day by minipumps did not block the secretory
response of the testes when incubated with hCG in vitro, or the
testosterone response to hCG injection in vivo. It is thus clear
that there are striking differences in the response to agonist
suppression even in the same species.

STUDIES IN DOGS

In female dogs during six months treatment with high doses of buserelin (up to 125 ug/kg daily s.c.), there was a marked involution
of the uterus and the ovaries (Sandow 1982a), associated with a significant decrease in plasma progesterone. During an 8 weeks post
treatment recovery period, plasma progesterone started to rise, and
the dogs developed functional corpora lutea. Studies on inhibition
of ovulation are not practical in female dogs because of the infre-
quent oestrous cycles, but the effects of agonists on follicular
oestrogen secretion can be tested. Pituitary suppression is evident
from the reduced LH response during agonist treatment. Male dogs

are very sensitive to agonist suppression. Either injections or continuous infusion will result in rapid lowering of plasma testosterone, together with involution of the testes and androgen-dependent
organs. In male dogs under high dose buserelin treatment (up to
125 ug/kg daily s.c. for 6 months), weight of the testes and prostate decreased greatly, associated with low plasma testosterone (Sandow et al. 1980). During an 8 weeks recovery period, testosterone
returned to pretreatment values, and the reproductive behaviour of
the dogs was restored to normal, when challenged with bitches in
heat. Treatment with peptide implants (125 ug/kg D-Trp^{6}LHRH(1-9)e-
thylamide) in beagle dogs was effective (after an initial stimulation phase) to lower plasma testosterone, and decrease prostate size within 36 days after implantation (Vickery 1981). The infusion
of buserelin 9 ug/kg/day at a constant rate from an implanted mini-
pump in a beagle dog leads to a marked decline of serum testosterone after 4 days, and values do not recover until the third day after infusion. In studies on suppression of spermatogenesis, a dose
of 10 ug/kg /D-(naphthyl-2)-Ala^6)LHRH (nafarelin) s. c. for 13 days
suppressed plasma testosterone, and reduced ejaculate volume, total
sperm count and motility score significantly for up to 50 days after treatment (Vickery 1981). The combination with testosterone implants which restituted plasma testosterone to low normal values
also reversed the antispermatogenic effect completely.

STUDIES IN PRIMATES

The evaluation of agonists and antagonists in primate species has
been a primary target of many investigators, because of the assumption that primates behave in a similar way as humans do. However,
significant differences to the clinical effects of agonists in humans are apparent in all primate species investigated so far. Generally, the sensitivity to agonist suppression is lower in monkeys,
and insensitivity of some species (bonnet monkeys) has been clai-
med. Female stumptail macaques (Macaca arctoides) require a higher
per kg dose than humans for suppression of ovulation (Fraser et al.
1980; Kerr-Wilson et al. 1981). In mature animals, a dose of 5 ug
buserelin daily s.c. suppressed ovulation in the majority of animals, but did not prevent intermittent oestradiol increases. Treatment for up to 400 days completely prevented luteal progesterone
increases. In some monkeys, the antiovulatory dose had to be raised
to 20 ug s.c./day for a consistent effect. The contraceptive effect
was rapidly reversible in all monkeys studied, ovulatory cycles
with appropriate progesterone increases occurred within 30 days after treatment. There was no secondary hormonal effects on thyroid
or adrenal function (Fraser 1983).

The cynomolgus monkey (Macaca fascicularis)is an interesting model
for testing agonist suppression of endometriosis. Recently, an effective treatment regimen with leuprolide, D-Leu^{6}LH-RH(1-9)ethylami-
de given by intermittent s.c. injection has been reported (Werlin &
Hodgen, 1983)), which however differs significantly from the effective regimen in women with endometriosis (Hardt & Schmidt-Gollwitzer, personal communication).

In male rhesus monkeys (Macaca mulatta), considerably higher doses
are required for inhibition of testicular function than in men. In
preclinical studies in men, a dose of 5 ug buserelin s.c. daily for
17 weeks reduced plasma testosterone to 50% of the initial values
(Bergquist et al. 1979a), whereas in rhesus monkeys, a daily dose
of 20 ug s.c for 4 weeks caused only a transient suppression of

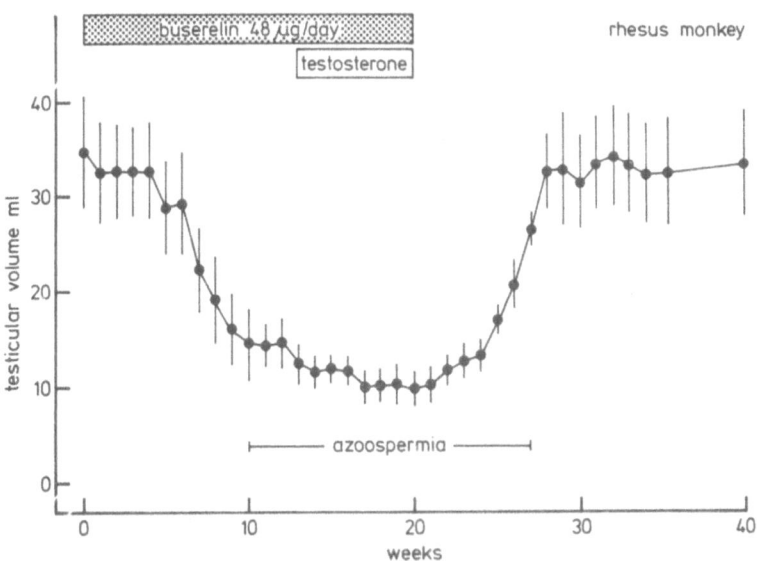

Fig. 1. Progress towards a male contraception: continuous infusion of an LHRH agonist, D-Ser(Bu^t)^{6}LHRH(1-9)ethylamide (buserelin) for 20 weeks in adult rhesus monkeys. Azoospermia developed after 10 weeks of infusion, and testosterone silastic implants restore spontaneous ejaculatory behaviour (Bint Akhtar et al., J. Clin. Endocrinol. Metab. $\underline{56}$, 534, 1983).

sperm counts (Wickings et al. 1981; Nieschlag et al. 1982). However, in the monkey a different type of suppression was highly effective. Constant subcutaneous infusion of buserelin from osmotic mini-pumps at a dose of 48 µg/day for 20 weeks resulted in pituitary desensitization with a loss of responsiveness to a test dose of 50 µg LHRH i.v. There was a rapid decrease of serum LH and testosterone to low levels, associated with a decrease in testicular volume. When the infusion was performed for 13 weeks, spontaneous ejaculation was completely suppressed, and azoospermia was found. After testosterone substitution from silastic implants, the ejaculatory behaviour was reestablished, but ejaculate size remained small and azoospermia persisted (Fig. 1). It was concluded, that constant infusion of the agonist is far more effective in male rhesus monkeys than daily injections and that the suppressive effects of agonist application are fully reversible (Bint Akhtar et al. 1983). It is therefore possible to use the primate model for the research on an LHRH-based male contraceptive, which requires testosterone substitution to restore ejaculation and reproductive behaviour. Treatment of rhesus monkeys with 500 µg D-Trp^{6}LHRH(1-9)ethylamide s.c. per day also reduced serum testosterone to low levels in two out of 4 monkeys pretreated with 500 µg of the agonist twice weekly for 19 weeks (Sundaram et al. 1981).

MECHANISM OF CONTRACEPTIVE ACTION

Although the contraceptive effects in male and female animals are
now firmly established, research on the several different mechanisms participating in a loss of pituitary and gonadal responsiveness
is a continuing effort, because these mechanisms are complex and
their relative importance in vivo is incompletely understood. Since
the primary hormone effect of agonists is to release LH and FSH in
supraphysiological quantities, investigation at the pituitary level
has focussed on pituitary responsiveness, and LHRH receptors. The
first conspicuous finding after repeated high dose injections of
LHRH or agonists is a diminishing LH release, finally leading to a
state of pituitary refractoriness. This process is time- and dose-
dependent and can be induced both in intact and castrate rats. In
gonadectomized animals, pituitary inhibition induced by agonists is
an LH-mediated phenomenon, which does not require the presence of
either gonadal or adrenal steroids (Sandow et al. 1978, 1979). A
short loop feedback of serum LH and FSH on pituitary secretion has
been established in the rabbit (Patritti-Laborde et al. 1979, 1981)
and in other species. Pituitary inhibition is also related to the
effect of agonists on pituitary LHRH receptors. At low doses, LHRH
receptors are induced (up-regulated), whereas at higher doses, they
are down-regulated to maintain a physiological optimum of secretion
(Clayton & Catt 1981; Clayton 1982). The characteristic pulsatile
pattern of LH secretion is easily disrupted by agonist injections,
even at low doses, due to the prolonged stimulation and receptor
occupancy. In pituitary cell cultures, pulsatile agonist administration gradually blocks LH release, in contrast to an equipotent dose
of LHRH (Yeo et al. 1982). A second mechanism for pituitary inhibition is desensitization by continuous infusion (Belchetz et al.
1978). During a prolonged LHRH infusion, LH increases temporarily,
followed by a progressive decline to basal levels. Pituitary desensitization to an LHRH infusion is observed in the human (Rabin and
McNeill 1980; Heber and Swerdloff 1981), and in experimental animals (Sandow 1982a, 1982b). Profound desensitization is achieved by
long-term infusion of LHRH agonists from osmotic minipumps implanted into the subcutaneous tissue (Sandow 1982b; Clayton 1982; Bint
Akhtar et al. 1983), or by peptide implants in the form of pellets
with delayed release (Vickery 1981). Desensitization is also observed in pituitary cell cultures, the reduced responsiveness can be
overcome by a supramaximal stimulatory dose of LHRH (Badger et al.
1983).

At the gonadal level, contraceptive action is due to three different mechanisms. Gonadotrophin receptors are down-regulated by excessive secretion of LH, a mechanism which induces dose-dependent
loss of LH- and prolactin-receptors, leading to testicular or ovarian involution or to luteolysis by inadequate luteal LH support.
The rapidity and magnitude of down-regulation depends on the suppressive dose of LHRH agonist administered. A second important mechanism is the change in steroid biosynthesis observed under agonist treatment. In male rats, the steroidogenic lesion consists of
a reduced activity of 17alpha-hydroxylase and 17,20-desmolase (Belanger et al. 1979; Labrie et al. 1980). Testosterone precursors
of low androgenic activity are preferentially secreted, and the
secretion of active androgens (testosterone, 5alpha-dihydrotestoste-
rone) is impaired. A third level for the action of LHRH agonists on
the reproductive system is related to direct interaction with gonadal binding sites for gonadotrophins (Hsueh and Jones 1981). The
direct gonadal effect appears to consist of an initial stimulation
phase (Popkin et al. 1983). In granulosa cell cultures, the subse-

quent inhibitory effect on oestrogen production is well correlated with the hormonal potency of agonist analogues (Hsueh et al. 1983). In hypophysectomized animals substituted with gonadotrophin injections, simultaneous agonist treatment inhibits LHRH receptors and the activation of steroidogenesis by gonadotrophins. The functional significance of these mechanisms in the human is not clear. Direct gonadal inhibition is usually observed at relatively high suppressive doses in animals, and thus may also contribute to the inhibition of gonadal function observed in the human.

The involvement of prostaglandins in inhibition of testicular function by agonists has been suggested (Isidori et al. 1983), due to increased PGF- and PGE-levels found in testicular homogenate after treatment. Luteolytic prostaglandins have a marked inhibitory effect on testosterone secretion and biosynthesis (Sandow et al. 1981b).

STUDIES WITH LHRH ANTAGONISTS

Antagonists bind to the pituitary LHRH receptor and block the action of endogenous LHRH. They are capable of selectively blocking secretion of LH and FSH without an initial stimulation phase, as observed with agonists. The structural development of LHRH antagonists (Rivier et al. 1981c; Schally et al. 1981) has resulted in highly active peptides, with extensive modification of the LHRH structure by substitutions in positions 1, 2, 3, 6 and 10, either by D-amino acids or halogenated D-amino acids. Test systems for antagonistic potency in rodents, and in primates have confirmed the possibility of using such peptides for the control of fertility (Asch et al. 1981; Balmaceda et al. 1982; Coy et al. 1982; Rivier et al. 1979, 1981a, 1981b). The future development of antagonists is particularly intriguing, because they may be orally active due to their multiple enzyme resistant substitutions. Oral activity has been confirmed in the rat (Nekola et al. 1982). It has been demonstrated, that antagonists can terminate pregnancy in rats (Rivier et al. 1979), and reversibly inhibit fertility in male rats (Rivier et al. 1981c). They are also capable of blocking ovulation in the human (Zarate et al. 1981). The evaluation of antagonists in primates is difficult because of the exact timing required for their administration. In rhesus monkeys, an oestradiol challenge can induce ovulation despite acute pituitary stalk section eliminating endogenous LHRH secretion (Ferin et al. 1979). Since in primates the preovulatory LH surge and ovulation can occur independently of an endogenous LHRH increase prior to ovulation, it will be necessary to administer antagonists for several days preceding ovulation to inhibit follicular maturation and block oestrogen secretion together with LHRH action. Hypothalamic activity is indispensible for follicular maturation in primates, long-term pituitary stalk section eventually leads to pituitary refractoriness to oestradiol stimulation.

Due to their different mode of action, antagonists offer an intriguing potential for contraceptive peptides of a type different from the agonists, but long-term reversibility of pituitary suppression may be a particular problem.

METABOLISM OF AGONISTS

The main advantages of using LHRH agonists for contraception are
favourable biological tolerance and highly specific hormone action.
Their suppressive effect is also rapidly reversible. This is in
part due to the fact, that agonists are rapidly metabolized by
endogenous exo- and endopeptidases (Sandow et al. 1981c; Sandow
and Clayton 1983). Similarly to LHRH, highly active agonists of
the LHRH(1-9)nonapeptide-ethylamide type or of the LHRH-decapep-
tide type are degraded by enzymes present in liver, kidney and
anterior pituitary. In our studies in rats, metabolic inactivation
of buserelin 60 min. after intravenous injection of a suppressive
dose of 125-I-labelled peptide in rats, no intact buserelin was
recovered from the main inactivating organs (liver and kidney).
Extraction of the metabolites, and subsequent identification by
thin layer chromatography, enzyme digestion with pyroglutamyl-pep-
tidase/chymotrypsin and binding to specific buserelin antisera
indicated that C-terminal metabolites are predominantly formed,
such as the buserelin(3-9)heptapeptide and (4-9)hexapeptide. In
the anterior pituitary of rats, a specific metabolite MI was found,
and identified as the buserelin(2-9)octapeptide, resulting from
degradation by pyroglutamyl-peptidase. The primary inactivation
step completely terminates biological activity, even at the high
suppressive doses used in agonist therapy of hormone-dependent
tumours (prostate and mammary carcinoma).

Studies on the metabolism and pharmacokinetics of agonists are
complicated by the minute doses used for contraception. The serum
level of immunoreactive agonist usually decreases rapidly and falls
to nondetectable levels. However, the urinary excretion of immunoreactive metabolites is a sensitive and reliable parameter of agonist absorption, and has been measured after contraceptive doses
given by nasal spray. At higher suppressive doses used for therapy
of endometriosis, serum levels are easily detectable, but also
decrease rapidly after subcutaneous injection. There is no direct
correlation between the serum level and the biological effect induced on pituitary gonadotrophin secretion. Pharmacokinetic measurement of agonist levels in serum, or urinary excretion of agonists
is of particular advantage in situations, where the pituitary response is greatly reduced or fully suppressed by high doses (Sandow
et al. 1981a).

Another advantage of using agonists for contraception is their
low antigenicity. In a variety of treatment protocol for precocious
puberty, contraception or hormone dependent tumours, no formation
of antibodies either against the agonist or against LHRH has been
observed (Fraser et al. 1983). Furthermore, antisera raised against
LHRH(1-9)-ethylamide peptides do not crossreact with endogenous
LHRH. It is therefore unlikely, that agonist antibodies would block
pituitary function.

CONTRACEPTION IN HUMANS

An important medical application of agonists may be their contraceptive use as a safe, effective and reversible method of suppressing ovulation. The experimental results in animals are extensive,
but cannot be extrapolated directly to the human. There are many
possible regimens and dosage forms for pituitary-ovarian inhibition during the follicular phase, at ovulation and during the lutal
phase (see review by Fraser 1981). The initial observation of de-

creasing pituitary responsiveness after consecutive agonist injections (Dericks-Tan et al. 1977; Wiegelmann et al. 1977) provided
a pharmacological basis for reversible inhibition of ovarian function. Daily administration of an agonist nasal spray was found to
be effective in suppressing ovulation, and preventing luteal progesterone increases (Nillius et al. 1978; Bergquist et al. 1979b,
1979c, 1982; Baumann et al. 1980; Schmidt-Gollwitzer et al. 1981a,
1981b, 1981c). This regimen has the advantage of simplicity, but
may induce amenorrhea or irregular bleeding. Subsequently, a variety of different approaches was tried with limited success. Administration early in the menstrual cycle may induce a deficient corpus
luteum due to insufficient FSH stimulation (Sheehan et al. 1982;
Skarin et al. 1982a). This approach depends critically on sufficient suppression of FSH secretion, which is not easily achieved. If
the peptide is administered throughout the follicular phase of the
cycle, follicular maturation is impaired or suppressed and ovulation does not take place. However, if treatment is stopped at any

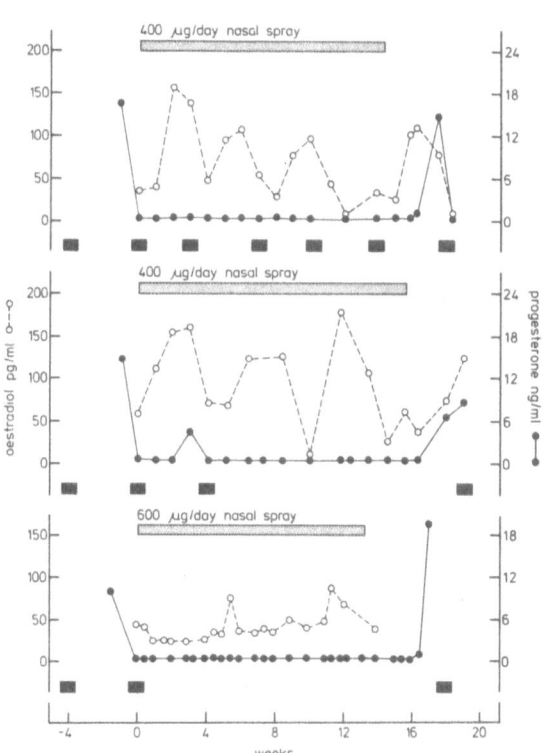

PEPTIDE CONTRACEPTION, CONTINUOUS ADMINISTRATION

Fig. 2. The contraceptive effect of daily agonist administration by
nasal spray (buserelin 400-600 μg). Plasma oestradiol and progesterone levels in three women treated for 93-109 days. Bleeding pattern indicated by squares (Bergquist et al., Clin. Endocrinol.
17:91, 1982).

time during the follicular phase, the menstrual cycle will only be shifted to a later onset with delayed ovulation, and a normal luteal phase (Hardt et al. 1982). To achieve a reliable contraceptive effect, the agonist has to be administered throughout the entire follicular phase to achieve pituitary desensitization and prevent the preovulatory LH release. The luteolytic approach, as indicated by the marked pre- and postcoital contraceptive effects of agonists in rats (Corbin and Bex 1981) has been investigated extensively in the human, and the luteal phase was found to be reduced during high dose agonist administration (Lemay et al. 1979a, 1979b, Casper and Yen 1979; Bergquist et al. 1980a). However, the luteolytic activity observed in animals has not been of practical importance, because the corpus luteum of pregnancy is protected by hCG from the effects of agonists on LH receptors (Bergquist et al. 1980b). There is no abortifacient effect of agonists during early pregnancy (Skarin et al. 1982b), or at 5-8 weeks of pregnancy (Tolis et al. 1982).

A practical method of contraception should be simple and easy to control. Since the time of ovulation cannot be anticipated with any certainty, agonists have to be administered from the first day of the follicular phase , but the difficulty of this approach is the absence of a luteal phase, if ovulation is suppressed. There is no secretory transformation of the endometrium by progesterone. In a discontinuous contraceptive regimen, a regular bleeding pattern can be established by the intermittent administration of a progestagen together with the agonist. In clinical studies with buserelin nasal spray (400-600 ug/day) without a progestagen, there was a wide range of bleeding patterns (Bergquist et al. 1981, 1982; Schmidt-Gollwitzer et al. 1981b, 1981c, Fig. 2). The wide range of individual reactions prompted the use of a cyclic contraceptive regimen, similarly to the use of sequential steroid preparations (Hardt et al. 1982). During the first phase of the contraceptive cycle, the peptide is adminstered by nasal spray for 21 days. On days 19-22, an orally active progestagen (norethisteron acetate 10 mg/day) is added to obtain secretory transformation of the endometrium (Fig. 3). The progestagen may also be administered at lower doses for 7 days to achieve a more physiological transformation, but side effects of the progestagen component will be more marked with this regimen.

The results of long term contraceptive studies indicate, that LHRH agonists provide reliable protection if administered throughout the menstrual cycle. The individual reaction to peptide suppression is monitored by progestagen administration, in a discontinuous regimen. A regular bleeding pattern indicates, that oestradiol has not been suppressed below physiological levels. Absence of bleeding after the progestagen is a symptom of agonist-induced amenorrhea. A pregnancy test should be performed to exclude contraceptive failures at this stage. Women suffering from moderate forms of hypothalamic amenorrhea may react with more rapid oestrogen suppression. In endometriosis and polycystic ovarian disease, high dose treatment is effective for a temporary block of oestradiol secretion and elevated ovarian androgens (Meldrum et al. 1982; Chang et al. 1983). Suppression of oestradiol secretion is also achieved in idiopathic precocious puberty (Comite et al. 1981).

The prospects for a male method based on a peptide contraceptive are difficult to evaluate. The biological advantages of agonists, namely their rapid reversibility and favourable biological tolerance justify further development. Daily administration appears to be required, or long-term treatment with sustained release pre-

PEPTIDE / PROGESTAGEN CONTRACEPTION

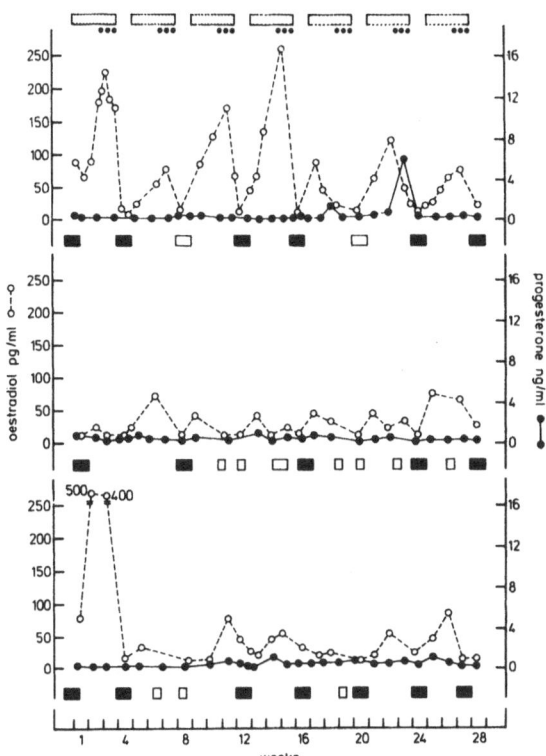

Fig. 3. Contraception by discontiunous administration of an LHRH agonist (buserelin nasal spray 400 µg once daily from days 1-22), together with a progestagen (circles) added on days 19-22. Plasma oestradiol and progesterone in three women treated for 28 weeks. Bleeding pattern indicated by open and closed boxes (Hardt et al., Geburtsh. u. Frauenheilk. 41:874, 1982).

parations. The disadvantage of a male peptide contraceptive is the requirement for androgen substitution, once azoospermia has been achieved (Bint Akhtar et al. 1983). Although inhibition of spermatogenesis has been observed in normal men with 50 µg D-Trp[6] LHRH(1-9)-ethylamide (Linde et al. 1981), the requirement for androgen substitution would make a male method difficult to control, because spermatogenesis can be re-established in some hypogonadal men by testosterone alone (Baranetsky and Carlson 1980).

30

SUMMARY

A new contraceptive method should be simple, safe and effective.
Furthermore, it should offer significant advantages in comparison
with existing methods. By these criteria, LHRH peptides have significant advantages with regard to highly specific hormonal action,
absence of side effects, favourable biological tolerance and rapid
reversibility of the contraceptive effects. LHRH agonists can be
administered daily, e.g. by nasal spray, and have been investigated
in sufficient detail to evaluate their potential. Ovulation is
reliably inhibited, and the absence of corpus luteum formation
requires intermittent and sequencial addition of a progestagen to
obtain endometrial transformation, and a regular bleeding pattern.
Other approaches have been unsuccessful, in particular early luteolysis, which is prevented by the hCG-increase of pregnancy. The
LHRH antagonists act via different mechanisms, blocking gonadotrophin secretion without an initial stimulation phase, and with less
marked changes at the gonadal level. The contraceptive efficacy of
peptide contraceptives will have to be studied in large field
trials as for any other new contraceptive method, they may provide
valuable alternatives to existing reversible methods of fertility
control.

ACKNOWLEDGMENT

The studies reported here are the result of collaborative work in
experimental endocrinology and clinical research. The authors would
like to thank Drs. H.M. Fraser, E. Nieschlag, S.J. Nillius, M.
Schmidt-Gollwitzer and W. Hardt for scientific discussion of specific topics covered in this review, and for kind permission to include illustrative material related to their studies. They would also
like to acknowledge the generous support of the National Institute
of Health, National Hormone and Pituitary Program, Maryland/USA,
and by Prof. A.F. Parlow.

REFERENCES

Asch, R.H., Balmaceda, J.P., Eddy, C.A., Siler-Khodr, T., Coy, D.H.
& Schally, A.V. (1981) Inhibition of the postcastration rise of luteinizing hormone and follicle-stimulating hormone in female rhesus
monkeys (Macaca mulatta) by the administration of a luteinizing hormone-releasing hormone inhibitory analog (/N-Ac-D-Trp[1,3],D-p-Cl-
Phe[2],D-Phe[6],D-Ala[10]/LH-RH). Fertil. Steril. 36:388-391

Badger, T.M., Loughlin, J.S. & Naddaff, P.G. (1983) The luteinizing
hormone-releasing hormone (LHRH)-desensitized rat pituitary: luteinizing hormone responsiveness to LHRH in vitro. Endocrinology
112:793-799

Balmaceda, J.P., Schally, A.V., Coy, D. & Asch, R.H. (1981) The ef-
fects of an LH-RH antagonist (/N-Ac-D-Trp[1,3],D-p-Cl-Phe[2],D-Phe[6],D-
Ala[10]/-LH-RH) during the preovulatory period of the rhesus monkey.
Contraception 24:275-281

Baranetsky, N.G. & Carlson, H.E. (1980) Persistence of spermatogenesis in hypogonadotropic hypogonadism treated with testosterone. The
American Fertility Society 34:477-482

Baumann, R., Kuhl, H., Taubert, H.D. & Sandow, J. (1980) Ovulation inhibition by daily i.m. administration of a highly active LH-RH analog (D-Ser(TBU)⁶-LH-RH(1-9)nonapeptide-ethylamide). Contraception 21:191-197

Belanger, A., Auclair, C., Ferland, L., Caron, S. & Labrie, F. (1980) Time-course of the effect of treatment with a potent LHRH agonist on tesicular steroidogenesis and gonadotropin receptor levels in the adult rat. J. Steroid Biochem. 13:191-196

Belchetz, P.E., Plant, T.M., Nakai, Y., Keogh, E.J. & Knobil, E. (1978) Hypophysial responses to continuous and intermittent delivery of hypothalamic gonadotropin-releasing hormone. Science 202:631-632

Bergquist, C., Nillius, S.J., Bergh, T., Skarin, G. & Wide, L. (1979a) Inhibitory effects on gonadotropin secretion and gonadal function in men during chronic treatment with a potent stimulatory luteinizing hormone-releasing hormone analogue. Acta Endocrinol. (Kbh.) 91:601-608

Bergquist, C., Nillius, S.J. & Wide, L. (1979b) Inhibition of ovulation in women by intranasal treatment with a luteinizing hormone-releasing hormone agonist. Contraception 19:497-506

Bergquist, C., Nillius, S.J. & Wide, L. (1979c) Intranasal gonadotropin-releasing hormone agonist as a contraceptive agent. Lancet II:215-217

Bergquist, C., Nillius, S.J. & Wide, L. (1980a) Effects of a luteinizing hormone-releasing hormone agonist on luteal function in women. Contraception 22:287-293

Bergquist, C., Nillius, S.J. & Wide, L. (1980b) Luteolysis induced by a luteinizing hormone-releasing hormone agonist is prevented by human chorionic gonadotropin. Contraception 22:341-347

Bergquist, C., Nillius, S.J., Wide, L. & Lindgren, A. (1981) Endometrial patterns in women on chronic luteinizing hormone-releasing hormone agonist treatment for contraception. Fertil. Steril. 36:339-342

Bergquist, C., Nillius, S.J. & Wide, L. (1982) Intranasal LHRH agonist treatment for inhibition of ovulation in women: clinical aspects. Clin. Endocrinol. 17:91-98

Bint Akhtar, F., Wickings, E.J., Zaidi, P. & Nieschlag, E. (1982) Pituitary and testicular function in sexually mature rhesus monkeys under high-dose LRH-agonist treatment. Acta Endocrinol. 101:113-118

Bint Akhtar, F., Marshall, G.R., Wickings, J. & Nieschlag, E. (1983) Reversible induction of azoospermia in rhesus monkeys by constant infusion of a gonadotropin-releasing hormone agonist using osmotic minipumps. J. Clin. Endocrinol. Metab. 56:534-540

Casper, R.F. & Yen, S.S.C. (1979) Induction of luteolysis in the human with a long-acting analog of luteinizing hormone-releasing factor. Science 204:408-410

Chang, R.J., Laufer, L.R., Meldrum, D.R., DeFazio, J., Lu, J.K.H., Vale, W.W., Rivier, J.E. & Judd, H.L. (1983) Steroid secretion in polycystic ovarian disease after ovarian suppression by a long-acting gonadotropin-releasing hormone agonist. J. Clin. Endocrinol. Metab. 56:897-903

Clayton, R.N. (1982) Gonadotropin-releasing hormone modulation of its own pituitary receptors: Evidence for biphasic regulation. Endocrinology 111:152-161

Clayton, R.N. & Catt, K.J. (1981) Gonadotropin-releasing hormone receptors: characterization, physiological regulation, and relationship to reproductive function. Endocr. Rev. 2:186-209

Corbin, A. & Bex, F.J. (1980) Luteinizing hormone releasing hormone and analogues: conceptive and contraceptive potential. In: Progress in Hormone Biochemistry and Pharmacology, Vol. 1 (eds. M. Briggs & A. Corbin) Eden Press, Westmount, Canada, pp. 227-297

Corbin, A. & Bex, F.J. (1981) Physiology and contraceptive effects of LHRH and agonistic analogs in female animals. In: LHRH Peptides as Female and Male Contraceptives, eds: G.I. Zatuchni, J.D. Shelton and J.J. Sciarra, PARFR Series on Fertility Regulation, Harper and Row, Philadelphia, pp. 321-336

Comite, F., Cutler Jr., G.B., Rivier, J., Vale, W.W., Loriaux, D.L., & Crowley Jr., W.F. (1981) Short-term treatment of idiopathic precocious puberty with a long-acting analogue of luteinizing hormone-releasing hormone. New Engl. J. Med. 305:1546-1550

Coy, D.H., Horvath, A., Nekola, M.V., Coy, E., Erchegyi, J. & Schally, A.V. (1982) Peptide antagonists of LH-RH: Large increases in antiovulatory activities produced by basic D-amino acids in the six position. Endocrinology 110:1445-1447

Cusan, L., Auclair, C., Belanger, A., Ferland, L., Kelly, P.A., Seguin, C. & Labrie, F. (1979) Inhibitory effects of long term treatment with a luteinizing hormone-releasing hormone agonist on the pituitary-gonadal axis in male and female rats. Endocrinology 104:1369-1376

DeFazio, J., Meldrum, D.R., Laufer, L., Vale, W., Rivier, J., Lu, J.K.H. & Judd, H.L. (1983) Induction of hot flashes in premenopausal women treated with a long-actin GnRH agonist. J. Clin. Endocrinol. Metab. 56:445-448

Dericks-Tan, J.S.E., Hammer, E. & Taubert, H.D. (1977) The effect of D-Ser(TBU)^{6}LH-RH-EA^{10} upon gonadotropin release in normally cyclic women. J. Clin. Endocrinol. Metab. 45:597-600

Ferin, M., Rosenblatt, H., Carmel, P.W., Antunes, J.L. & Vande Wiele, R.L. (1979) Estrogen-induced gonadotropin surges in female rhesus monkeys after pituitary stalk section. Endocrinology 104:50-52

Fraser, H.M. (1981) Luteinizing hormone releasing hormone and fertility control. In: Oxford Reviews of Reproductive Biology, Vol. 3 (ed. C.A. Finn), Clarendon Press, Oxford, pp. 1-48

Fraser, H.M. (1983) Effect of treatment for 1 year with a luteinizing hormone-releasing hormone agonist on ovarian, thyroidal, and adrenal function and menstruation in the stumptailed monkey (Macaca arctoides). Endocrinology 112:245-253

Fraser, H.M., Laird, N.C. & Blakeley, D.M. (1980) Decreased pituitary responsiveness and inhibition of the luteinizing hormone surge and ovulation in the stumptailed monkey (Macaca arctoides) by chronic treatment with an agonist of luteinizing hormone-releasing hormone. Endocrinology 106:452-457

Fraser, H.M., Sharpe, R.M., Lincoln, G.A. & Harmer, A.J. (1982) LH-RH antibodies: Their use in the study of hypothalamic LHRH and testicular LHRH-like material, and possible contraceptive applications. In: Progress Towards a Male Contraceptive, eds: S.L. Jeffcoate and M. Sandler, John Wiley & Sons, London, pp. 41-78

Fraser, H.M., Sandow, J. & Krauss, B. (1983) Antibody production against an agonist analogue of luteinizing hormone-releasing hormone: Evaluation of immunochemical and physiological consequences. Acta Endocrinologica, in press

Hardt, W., Schmidt-Gollwitzer, K., Nevinny-Stickel, J. & Schmidt-Gollwitzer, M. (1982) Fortschritte in der kontrazeptiven Anwendung des LHRH Agonisten Buserelin: Diskontinuierliche Medikation mit gestageninduzierter Abbruchblutung (Progress in contraceptive application of the LHRH agonist, buserelin: discontinuous medication with progestogen-induced withdrawal bleeding). Geburtshilfe Frauenheilkd. 42:874-877

Heber, D. & Swerdloff, R.S. (1981) Down-regulation of pituitary gonadotropin secretion in postmenopausal females by continuous gonadotropin-releasing hormone administration. J. Clin. Endocrinol. Metab. 52:171-172

Hsueh, A.J.W. & Jones, P.B.C. (1981) Extrapituitary actions of gonadotropin-releasing hormone. Endocr. Rev. 2:437

Hsueh, A.J.W., Adashi, E.Y., Tucker, E., Valk, C. & Ling, N.C. (1983) Relative potencies of gonadotropin-releasing hormone agonists and antagonists on ovarian and pituitary functions. Endocrinology 112:689-695

Isidori, A., Conte, D., Spera, G., Toscano, V., Citarella, F., Paolucci, D., Foli, S., Stigliani, V., Boniforti, L. & Betto, B. (1983) Possible involvement of prostaglandins in GnRH action at testicular level. In: Recent Advances in Male Reproduction, ed.: R. D'Agata, Raven Press, New York, in press

Kerr-Wilson, R.H.J., MacKenzie, L. & Fraser, H.M. (1981) Effects of chronic LHRH agonist treatment on the endometrium and ovaries of the stump-tailed macaque. Contraception 24:647-655

Knobil, E. (1980) The neuroendocrine control of the menstrual cycle. Recent Prog. Horm. Res. 36:53-88

Labrie, F., Belanger, A., Cusan, L., Seguin, C., Pelletier, G., Kelly, P.A., Reeves, J.J., Lefebvre, F.A., Lemay, A., Gourdeau, Y. & Raynaud, J.P. (1980) Antifertility effects of LH-RH agonists in the male. J. Androl. 1:209-227

Lemay, A., Labrie, F., Ferland, L. & Raynaud, J.P. (1979a) Possible luteolytic effects of luteinizing hormone-releasing hormone in normal women. Fertil. Steril. 31:29-34

Lemay, A., Labrie, F., Belanger, A. & Raynaud, J.P. (1979b) Luteolytic effect of intranasal administration of (D-Ser(TBU)^6,des-Gly-HN$_2$^{10})-luteinizing hormone-releasing hormone ethylamide in normal women. Fertil. Steril. 32:646-651

Linde, R., Doelle, G.C., Alexander, N., Kirchner, F., Vale, W., Rivier, J. & Rabin, D. (1981) Reversible inhibition of testicular steroidogenesis and spermatogenesis by a potent gonadotropin-releasing hormone agonist in normal men. New Engl. J. Med. 305:663-667

Meldrum, D.R., Chang, R.J., Lu, J., Vale, W., Rivier, J. & Judd, H.L. (1982) "Medical oophorectomy" using a longacting GnRH agonist - a possible new approach to the treatment of endometriosis. J. Clin. Endocrinol. Metab. 54:1081-1083

Nekola, M.V., Horvath, A., Ge, L.J., Coy. D.H. & Schally, A.V. (1982) Suppression of ovulation in the rat by an orally active antagonist of luteinizing hormone-releasing hormone. Science 218:160-162

Nieschlag, E., Akhtar, F.B., Marshall, G.R. & Wickings, E.J. (1982) The rhesus monkey as an experimental model for therapeutic application of LHRH and its analogues. In: Therapy in Andrology, eds: G.F. Menchini-Fabris, W. Pasini and L. Martini, Excerpta Medica, Amsterdam, International Congress Series 596, pp. 108-114

Nillius, S.J., Bergquist, C. & Wide, L. (1978) Inhibition of ovulation in women by chronic treatment with a stimulatory LRH analogue - a new approach to birth control? Contraception 17:537-545

Patritti-Laborde, N., Wolfsen, A., Heber, D. & Odell, W.D. (1979) Pituitary gland: site of shortloop feedback for luteinizing hormone in the rabbit. J. Clin. Invest. 64:1066

Patritti Laborde, N., Wolfsen, A.R. & Odell, W.D. (1981) Short loop feedback system for the control of follicle-stimulating hormone in the rabbit. Endocrinology 108:72-75

Popkin, R., Fraser, H.M. & Jonassen, J. (1983) Stimulation of androstenedione and progesterone release by LHRH and LHRH agonist from isolated rat preovulatory follicles. Mol. Cell. Endocrinol. 29:169-179

Puri, C.P. & Csapo, A.I. (1981) Evaluation of antifertility effects of LHRH analogs in the guinea pig. In: LHRH Peptides as Female and Male Contraceptives, eds.: G.I. Zatuchni, J.D. Shelton & J.J. Sciarra, Harper & Row, Philadelphia, pp. 126-133

Rabin, D. & McNeill, L.W. (1980) Pituitary and gonadal desensitization after continuous luteinizing hormone-releasing hormone infusion in normal females. J. Clin. Endocrinol. Metab. 51:873-876

Rivier, C., Rivier, J. & Vale, W. (1979) Effect of the LRF-antagonist (D-pGlu^1,D-Phe^2,D-Trp^{3,6})-LRF on pregnancy in the rat. Contraception 19:185-190

Rivier, C., Rivier, J. & Vale, W. (1981 a) Antireproductive effects of a potent GnRH antagonist in the female rat. Endocrinology 108:1425-1430

Rivier, C., Rivier, J. & Vale, W. (1981 b) Effect of a potent GnRH antagonist and testosterone propionate on mating behaviour and fertility in the male rat. Endocrinology 108, 1998-2001

Rivier, C., Rivier, J. & Vale, W.W. (1981c). GnRH antagonists: Physiologic and contraceptive applications in the female rat. In LHRH Peptides as Female and Male Contraceptives, eds.: G.I. Zatuchni, J.D. Shelton and J.J. Sciarra, Harper & Row, Philadelphia, pp. 140-150

Sandow, J. (1982a) Gonadotropic and antigonadotropic actions of LH-RH analogues. In: Neuroendocrine Perspectives, Vol. 1, eds.: E.E. Müller & R.M. McLeod, Elsevier Biomedical Press, Amsterdam, pp. 339-395

Sandow, J. (1982b) Inhibition of pituitary and testicular function by LHRH analogues. In: Progress Towards a Male Contraceptive, eds.: S.L. Jeffcoate & M. Sandler, John Wiley and Sons, London, pp. 19-39

Sandow, J. (1983) Clinical applications of LHRH and its analogues. Clin. Endocrinol. 18:571-592

Sandow, J. & Clayton, R.N. (1983) The disposition, metabolism, kinetics and receptor binding properties of LHRH and its analogues. In: Progress in Hormone Biochemistry and Pharmacology, Vol. 2, Eden Press, London, in press

Sandow, J., Rechenberg, W.v., Jerzabek, G. & Stoll, W. (1978) Pituitary gonadotropin inhibition by a highly active analogue of LH-RH. Fertil. Steril. 30:205-209

Sandow, J., Rechenberg, W.v., Kuhl, H., Baumann, R., Krauss, B., Jerzabek, G. & Kille, S. (1979) Inhibitory control of the pituitary LH secretion by LH-RH in male rats. Hormone Res. 11:303-317

Sandow, J., Rechenberg, W. v., Baeder, C. & Engelbart, K. (1980) Antifertility effects of an LHRH analogue in male rats and dogs. Intern. J. Fertil. 25:213-221

Sandow, J., Clayton, R.N. & Kuhl, H. (1981a) Pharmacology of LH-RH and its analogues. In: Endocrinology of Human Infertility: New Aspects, eds.: P. Crosignani and B.L. Rubin, Academic Press, London, pp. 221-246

Sandow, J., Rechenberg, W.v., Hahn, M. & Kille, S. (1981b) Experimentelle Prüfung luteolytischer Prostaglandine. In: Prostaglandine in Gynäkologie und Geburtshilfe, eds: H. Hepp and B. Schüßler, Springer Verlag, Berlin, pp. 52-61

Sandow, J., Jerabek-Sandow, G., Krauss, B. & Stoll, W. (1981c) Metabolic and dispositional studies with LHRH analogs. In: LHRH Peptides as Female and Male Contraceptives, eds.: G.I. Zatuchni, J.D. Shelton & J.J. Sciarra, Harper & Row, Philadelphia, pp. 321-336

Schally, A.V., Arimura, A. & Coy, D.H. (1981) Recent approaches to fertility control based on derivatives of LH-RH. Vitam. Horm. 38:257-310

Schmidt-Gollwitzer, M., Hardt, W., Schmidt-Gollwitzer, K. & Nevinny-Stickel, J. (1981a) Chronic treatment with a LHRH agonist: a new contraceptive method? Acta Europ. Fertil. 12:175-276

Schmidt-Gollwitzer, M., Hardt, W., Schmidt-Gollwitzer, K. & Nevinny-Stickel, J. (1981b) Influence of the LH-RH analogue buserelin on cyclic ovarian function and on endometrium. A new approach to fertility control? Contraception 23:187-196

Schmidt-Gollwitzer, M., Hardt, W., Schmidt-Gollwitzer, K. & von der Ohe, M. (1981c) The contraceptive use of buserelin, a potent LH-RH agonist: clinical and hormonal findings. In: LHRH Peptides as Female and Male Contraceptives, eds.: G.I. Zatuchni, J.D. Shelton & J.J. Sciarra, Harper & Row, Philadelphia, pp. 199-215

Sheehan, K.L., Casper, R.F. & Yen, S.S.C. (1982) Luteal phase defects induced by an agonist of luteinizing hormone-releasing factor: a model for fertility control. Science 215:170-172

Skarin, G., Nillius, S.J. & Wide, L. (1982a) Early follicular phase luteinizing hormone-releasing hormone agonist administration - effects on follicular maturation and corpus luteum function in women. Contraception 25:31-39

Skarin, G., Nillius, S.J. & Wide, L. (1982b) Failure to induce abortion of early human pregnancy by high doses of a superactive LRH agonist. Contraception 26:457-463

Sundaram, K., Wang, N.G. & Bardin, C.W. (1981) Antigonadal, antisteroidal, and antifertility effects of LHRH agonists in male animals. In: LHRH Peptides as Female and Male Contraceptives, eds.: G.I. Zatuchni, J.D. Shelton & J.J. Sciarra, pp. 261-274, Harper & Row, Philadelphia

Tolis, G., Mehta, A.E., Schally, A.V., Comaru-Schally, A.M., Haber, G., Yufe, B., Popkin, D. & Kinch, R. (1982a) Failure to interrupt established pregnancy in humans by D-tryptophan 6-LHRH. Fertil. Steril. 36:241-242

Vickery, B.H. (1981) Physiology and antifertility effects of LHRH and agonistic analogs in male animals. In: LHRH Peptides as Female and Male Contraceptives, eds: G.I. Zatuchni, J.D. Shelton and J.J. Sciarra, Harper & Row, Philadelphia, pp. 275-290

Werlin, L.B. & Hodgen, G.D. (1983) Gonadotropin-releasing hormone agonist suppresses ovulation, menses and endometriosis in monkeys: An individualized, intermittent regimen. J. Clin. Endocrinol. Metab. 56:844-848

Wickings, E.J., Zaidi, P. & Nieschlag, E. (1981) Effects of chronic, high-dose LHRH-agonist treatment on pituitary and testicular functions in rhesus monkeys. J. Androl. 2:72-79

Wiegelmann, W., Solbach, H.G., Kiley, H.K. & Kruskemper, H.L. (1977) LH and FSH response to long-term application of LH-RH analogue in normal males. Horm. Metab. Res. 9:521-522

Yen, S.S.C. (1983) Clinical applications of gonadotropin-releasing hormone and gonadotropin-releasing hormone analogs. Fertil. Steril. 39:257-266

Yeo, T., Grossman, A., Belchetz, P. & Besser, G.M. (1982) Response of luteinizing hormone from columns of dispersed rat pituitary cells to a highly potent analogue of luteinizing hormone releasing hormone. J. Endocrinol. 91:33-41

Zarate, A., Canales, E.S., Sthory, I., Coy, D.H., Comaru-Schally, A.M. & Schally, A.V. (1981) Anovulatory effect of a LHRH antagonist in women. Contraception 24:315-320

Pulsatile Administration of Gn-RH in Hypothalamic Amenorrhea

G. Leyendecker and L. Wildt

Department of Obstetrics and Gynecology, University of Bonn, D-5300 Bonn

INTRODUCTION

Gonadotropin relaesing-hormone (Gn-RH) was the second of the neurohumoral agents postulated by Harris more than three decades ago to mediate hypothalamic control of anterior pituitary function that has been isolated, identified in its structure and synthesized. Since this was achieved by the groups of Schally and Guillemin in 1971 and the synthetic hormone became available, Gn-RH has been used extensively as tool in neuroendocrine research. Early attempts to use this decapeptide clinically for the treatment of reproductive disorders supposed to be due to an inadequate secretion of endogenous Gn-RH, however, were of only limited success. Effective therapeutic use had to await further progress in the understanding of the physiologic significance of pulsatile gonadotropin secretion and gonadal function. The demonstration that the pattern of the hypophysiotropic stimulation is of critical importance in this respect and the elucidation of the physiologic significance of pulsatile Gn-RH secretion have provided the rational basis for the efficient use of synthetic Gn-RH in the treatment of Gn-RH deficiency. These findings have also furthered the understanding of the seemingly paradoxical antifertility effects of long acting Gn-RH analogues initially designed to compensate for the short action of the parent decapeptide and thus to simplify treatment of infertility. In this communication, following a short review on physiologic and pathophysiologic aspects of hypothalamic control of gonadotropin secretion in the human female, clinical data obtained with chronic-intermittent (pulsatile) administration of Gn-RH in hypothalamic amenorrhea (HA) will be presented.

THE PULSATILE PATTERN OF GONADOTROPIN SECRETION DURING THE NORMAL MENSTRUAL CYCLE

The pattern of gonadotropin secretion during the normal menstrual cycle is characterized by low serum levels of LH and FSH during the follicular and luteal phases of the cycle interrupted by a sharp increase of LH and FSH during midcycle which causes ovulation. It has been shown by numerous investigators that this cyclic pattern of pituitary gonadotropin secretion can be regarded as a result of negative and positive feedback effects of ovarian steroids on pituitary function (Knobil, 1980; Leyendecker and Wildt, 1983a).

As first demonstrated in the castrated rhesus monkey, the pituitary release of LH is pulsatile in nature reflecting a pulsatile stimulation of the pituitary gonadotrophs by hypothalamic Gn-RH (Dierschke et al., 1970). By measurement of immunoreactive Gn-RH in the portal stalk effluent (Carmel et al., 1976) and in the cerebrospinal fluid of the third ventricle (Van Vugt et al., 1983) of the rhesus monkey direct evidence for the secretory pattern of hypothalmic Gn-RH could be provided. The pulsatile secretion of Gn-RH is directed by the arcuate nucleus of the mediobasal hypothalamus (Knobil, 1980). Selective destruction of this region in the brain

will abolish pituitary secretion of LH and FSH. Moreover, electrophysiological
studies have shown that rhythmic increases in multiunit activity in the region
of the arcuate nucleus are coincident with the initiation of LH pulses in
serum (Knobil, 1981).

In the agonadal female high amplitude LH pulses are observed every 90 minutes
on the average (Yen et al., 1982; Santen and Bardin, 1973). The same studies had
established that pulses with approximately this frequency, but a lower amplitude
occur during the follicular phase of the cycle, while during the luteal phase low-
frequency-high-amplitude pulses prevail. A more close analysis of the pulsatile
pattern of the LH release revealed that from day 3 - 5 of the follicular phase
until after the midcycle surge pulse frequency does not change and is maintained at
one pulse every 9o minutes (Leyendecker and Wildt, 1983a; Wildt et al., 1983).
During the luteal phase there is a progressive decline in LH pulse frequency,
which is lowest immediately before menstruation and increases again during the first
few days of early follicular phase. There is no direct relationship between progesterone concentrations and the reduction in LH pulse frequency. The reduction, however, appears to be correlated with the duration of the progesterone elevation.
The physiologic significance of the changing frequency of gonadotropin secretion
during the menstrual cycle, particularly during the luteal phase, remains to be
elucidated. The observation that normal menstrual cycles can be induced in women
Leyendecker et al., 1980a, 1981) and in rhesus monkeys (Knobil, 1980) with essentially abolished endogenous Gn-RH secretion by the pulsatile administration of
Gn-RH at an unvarying frequency, however, argues strongly against any major physiologic importance of this phenomenon for the regulation of luteal function and of
follicular development.

PATTERN OF GONADOTROPIN SECRETION IN PATIENTS WITH HYPOTHALAMIC AMENORRHEA

Complete absence or severe reduction of pulsatile gonadotropin release results
in impairment of follicular maturation, anovulation and amenorrhea (Leyendecker,
1979; Leyendecker et al., 1981). While this obtains physiologically before puberty
or during pregnancy and lactation, it is pathological in other periods of reproductive life. Since there is substantial indirect evidence that cause of this kind of
amenorrhea is a reduced stimulation of the anterior pituitary gland by Gn-RH and since
Gn-RH is secreted from the hypothalamus, it is referred to as hypothalamic amenorrhea
(Leyendecker, 1979; Leyendecker and Wildt, 1983b).

The term "hypothalamic amenorrhea" was coined by Klinefelter and associates in 1943
to describe amenorrhea of suprapituitary origin. Due to some cases described in the
original publication, however, it was later on confined to psychogenic amenorrhea.
In this communication, hypothalamic amenorrhea is used in its broader original sense
and consequently applies for patients with lesions of the pituitary stalk or hypothalamus, anorexia nervosa, Kallmann's syndrome as well as for idiopathic or psychogenic amenorrhea.

Since endogenous Gn-RH cannot be measured reliably in peripheral blood direct evaluation of hypothalamic function is presently not possible. Therfore, the diagnosis
of hypothalamic amenorrhea is essentially based on the exclusion of other causes
of amenorrhea, such as hyperprolactinemia, hyperandrogenemia, primary ovarian
failure, genital tract defects as well as internal and neurological diseases.
Primary pituitary failure is excluded by the ability to stimulate pituitary gonadotropic function by pulsatile administration of Gn-RH.

Based on studies in amenorrhoic patients, prepubertal subjects and experimental animals
the view has been advanced that hypothalamic amenorrhea forms a pathophysiological

continuum, reflecting a gliding scale of impairment of hypothalamic Gn-RH secretion and consequently gonadotropin production and follicular development and it was furthermore proposed that the extent of this impairment can be assessed by the response to Gn-RH-, gestagen-, and clomiphene-administration (Leyendecker, 1979; Leyendecker and Wildt, 1983b). The reactions in those simple tests have therefor been used as criteria for grading of amenorrhoic patients according to the severity of hypothalamic impairment and for selection of the appropriate therapy (table 1).

Table 1. Grading of hypothalamic amenorrhea on the basis of clomiphene-. gestagen- and Gn-RH-tests, respectively

Grade	Result of test
1	Clomiphene positive (bleeding)
2	Gestagen positive (bleeding) Clomiphene negative (no bleeding)
3	Gestagen negative (no bleeding) with pituitary response to 100 µg of Gn-RH i.v.
3a	"adult" response
3b	"prepubertal" response
3c	no response

Recent studies on the pulsatile pattern of LH in serum (figure 1), the frequency of LH pulses, overall LH and FSH levels during a 24 hour period as well as on ultrasonographic visualization of ovarian follicles in 20 patients suffering from hypothalamic amenorrhea supported this view (figure 2) (Wildt et al., 1983). The number of LH pulses was lowest in grade 3c patients and increased gradually until a value comparable of that of the normal menstrual cycle was reached in grade 2 patients. Only in garde 3b patients an increase in pulse frequency during sleep became apparent, while in all other grades pulses were found to be evenly distribu- ted between sleep and awake periods. Amplitude of some LH pulses, however, was considerably larger during sleep than during awake periods in grade 3b, 3a and grade 2 subjects. Overall LH and FSH levels increased parallel to the number of LH pulses up to grade 3a and 2, respectively, but failed to reach values typical for the early follicular phase of the cycle. In clomiphene positive patients, LH and parti- cularly FSH levels declined again and this may be attributed to negative feedback inhibition by the elevated levels of estradiol found in those patients.

Considerable follicular development up to large antral stage has been found in ovarian biopsies of amenorrhoic patients (Nakano et al., 1982). This was reflected by the number of follicles identified by ultrasound, which increased parallel to the number of LH pulses from essentially undetectable in grade 3c patients to a hight comparable to that found during the phase of maximal follicular development during the early follicular phase of the cycle in clomiphene positive patients. Thus, hypothalamic amenorrhea is characterized by a reduced frequency and amplitude of gonadotropin secretion which is reflected by the concomitant reduction of ovarian follicular growth. In this context, a reduction of frequency of pulsatile gonadotro- pin secretion is distinctive for the most severe grades of hypothalamic amenorrhea, while a reduction in amplitude characterizes less pronounced grades of this disorder.

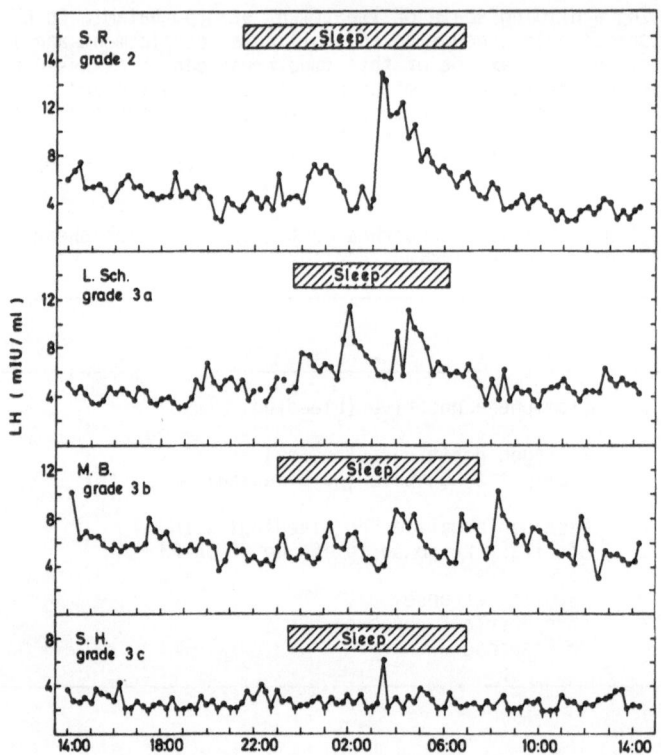

Fig. 1. Composite of the 24-hour secretory pattern of LH in representative patients suffering from different grades of hypothalamic amenorrhea, grading from virtually absent pulses in grade 3c to frequent pulsations with sleep-related increase in amplitude in grade 2. Vertical lines underneath data points indicate levels below assay sensitivity. From Leyendecker G, Wildt L (1983b), with permission.

One is tempted to speculate that the reduction of frequency and amplitude of pulsatile gonadotropin secretion closely reflects a corresponding reduction of frequency and amplitude of hypothalamic Gn-RH secretion, but this has still to await experimental proof. In any event, the findings provided by these investigations stronly support the earlier view that hypothalamic amenorrhea forms a pathophysiological continuum on the basis of a reduced Gn-RH secretion (Leyendecker, 1979; Leyendecker and Wildt, 1981, 1983b). They furthermore demonstrate, by showing a close correlation between the secretory pattern of gonadotropins and the results of the Gn-RH- (figure 3), gestagen- and clomiphene tests the validity of the grading system based on these tests and therefore support its use for the assessment of residual hypothalamic function in patients suffering from hypothalamic amenorrhea.

The pattern of gonadotropin secretion in patients suffering from different grades of hypothalamic amenorrhea closely resembles that observed during the developmental process of puberty (Boyar et al., 1972; Weitzman et al., 1975). At least from a descriptive point of view, hypothalamic amenorrhea may therefore be viewed as a

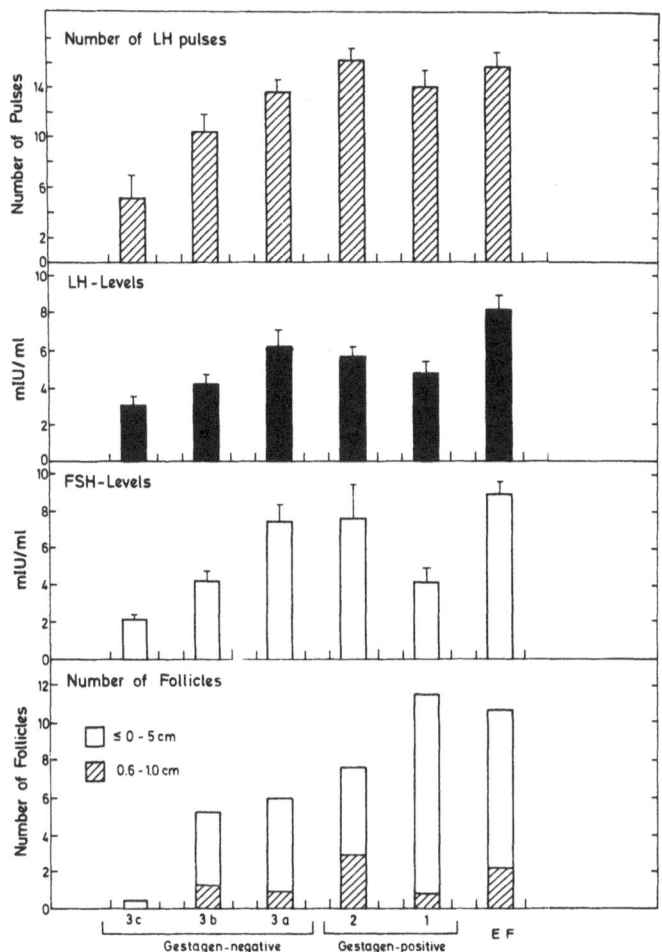

Fig. 2. Composite showing number of LH pulses in 24 hours, mean LH and FSH levels of the 24-hour sampling period and number of class I and class II follicles in patients suffering from hypothalamic amenorrhea graded according to response to Gn-RH-, gestagen- and clomiphene-administration. Bars indicate mean + SEM. The corresponding values for the early follicular phase (day 3 - 7) of 13 normal menstrual cycles (EF) are given for comparison and represent values of 8-hour sampling periods. The number of follicles given under EF represents the maximum number observed for each class of follicles . From Wildt et al. (1983), with permission.

regression into puberty or prepuberty in patients suffering from secondary amenorrhea, or as an arrest of the developmental process in those presenting with the primary form of this disorder. Such a mechanism has already been proposed for development of amenorrhea in anorexia nervosa (Boyar et al., 1974; Katz et al., 1977) but seems to apply for other forms of hypothalamic amenorrhea also.

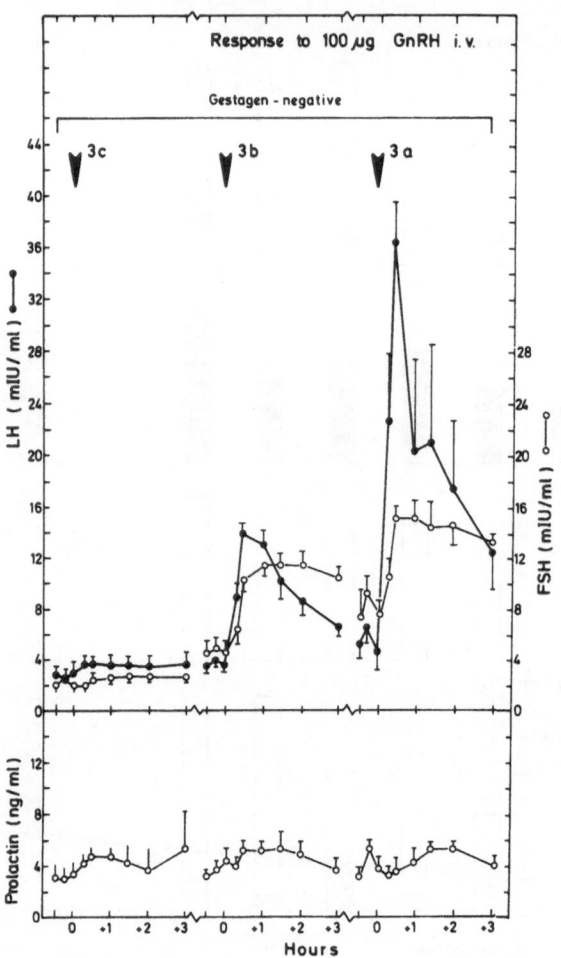

Fig. 3. Pituitary response to the i.v. injection of 100 µg Gn-RH in 13 gestagen negative patients with hypothalamic amenorrhea. Note the three clearly distinguishable response patterns: no response (grade 3c), prepubertal (grade 3b) and adult (grade 3a) response of LH and FSH. Each point represents mean + SEM of 4 (3a), 6 (3b) and 3 (3a) observations, respectively. From Leyendecker and Wildt (1983b) with permission.

THE FUNCTIONAL ROLE OF THE HYPOTHALAMUS IN THE REGULATION OF GONADOTROPIN SECRETION

The physiological significance of the pulsatile pattern of Gn-RH secretion did not become apparent until recently, when it was shown that only pulsatile and not conti- nuous administration of Gn-RH was able to maintain pituitary gonadotropic function in ovariectomized rhesus monkeys, in which endogenous Gn-RH secretion had been abo- lished by lesions in the medio-basal hypohalamus (Belchetz et al., 1980). The requirement of a pulsatile stimulation with Gn-RH by the pituitary gonadotrophs may explain, why administration of long acting analogues of the decapeptide was essentially unsuccessful in the treatment of secondary amenorrhea (Katzorke et al.,

1980) and did even deterioriate pituitary gonadotropic function in normal women
(Derick-Tan et al., 1977; Bergquist et al., 1979). Moreover, it could be demonstrated with the model of the hypothalamus lesioned rhesus monkey that the site of
action of estradiol in exhibiting negative and positive feedback effects on the
pituitary secretion of LH and FSH is localized on the level of the pituitary rather
than on the level of the brain (Nakai et al., 1978). In hypothalamus lesioned but
otherwise intact female rhesus monkeys the pulsatile administration of an unvarying
amount of Gn-RH at a physiologic frequency induced menstrual cycles which were not
different from spontaneous ones (Knobil et al., 1980). Thus, the endocrine regulation of the menstrual cycle of primates appears to be fundamentally different
from that of the estrous cycle of the rat. While in the rat the rostral part of the
hypothalamus seems to be essential in the mediation of chrono-biological signals
and positive feedback reactions, the assumption of such a "cyclic center" appears
no longer to be justified for the primate. In the primate the function of the hypothalamus in the regulation of the menstrual cycle is only a "permissive" one
(Knobil et al., 1980).

In women with severe hypothalamic amenorrhea, a condition functionally comparable
with that of the hypothalamus lesioned female rhesus monkey, chronic intermittent
(pulsatile) administration of Gn-RH with an unvarying dose and at an unchanged
frequency of one pulse every 90 minutes resulted in follicular maturation, ovulation and corpus luteum formation (Leyendecker, 1979; Leyendecker et al., 1980a).
the endocrine pattern of the normal menstrual cycle could be completely replicated.

Thus, it could be shown that the concept of the permissive function of the hypothalamus developed in the rhesus monkey could be extended to the human female.
These results have been confirmed by other investigators (Crowley and McArthur,
1980; Keogh et al., 1981; Schoemaker et al., 1982; Skarin et al., 1982) and with
the development of chronic-intermittent (pulsatile) administration of Gn-RH by
means of a small computerized pump ("Zyklomat", Ferring GmbH, Kiel, FRG) as a new
and practical mode of treatment of infertility in hypothalamic amenorrhea clinical advantage has been taken of these new insights into the physiology of the
human menstrual cycle (Leyendecker et al., 1980b; Leyendecker and Wildt, 1981, 1983b).

CLINICAL RESULTS OF PULSATILE ADMINISTRATION OF GN-RH IN HYPOTHALAMIC AMENORRHEA

Since the first introduction of pulsatile administration of Gn-RH to women with
hypothalamic amenorrhea 130 experimental and treatment cycles hace so far been
performed in our institution. The patients were selected for pulsatile treatment
on the basis of the criteria described above. Only patients with hypothalamic
amenorrhea of grades 2 - 3c were considered suitable for Gn-RH substitution.

Dose of Gn-RH

Intravenous administration of Gn-RH with a dose of 10 µg per pulse did not result
in full follicular maturation over a treatment period of 17 days in a patient with
primary hypothalamic amenorrhea grade 3c (Leyendecker et al., 1980a). The same
patient did however ovulate and exhibit normal luteal phases repeatedly when i.v.
doses of 15 - 20 µg/pulse were used. Doses of 2.5 and 5 µg/pulse again resulted
only in anovulatory bleeding (Leyendecker et al., 1981). In contrast, women with
hypothalamic amenorrhea grades 3b, 3a and 2, respectively, ovulated with i.v.
doses ranging from 2.5 - 20 µg/pulse, indicating that in less severe cases than
grade 3c a smaller dose of Gn-RH might be sufficient to induce menstrual cycles.
However, in these patients a dose of 1 - 2,5 µg/pulse might constitute a critical
dose range for induction of ovulation. In a patient with secondary hypothalamic
amenorrhea garde 2 with a dose of 1 µg/pulse ovulation could not be induced over
a treatment period of 41 days. When the dose was increased to 5 µg/pulse ovulation
was obtained and the patient conceived during that treatment course. As a consequence
of these findings, patients with hapothalamic amenorrhea grade 3c (usually patients

with primary amenorrhea or pituitary stalk and hypothalamic lesions exhibit this
degree of severity) are now routinely treated with 15 - 20 µg/pulse and the less
serious cases with 5 µg/pulse when the i.v. route is used. With this dose regimen
of Gn-RH all i.v. treatment cycles performed so far resulted in ovulation.

Once the critical threshold of the Gn-RH dose is surpassed there seems to be
a dose response relationship between the dose of Gn-RH administered per pulse and
the ovarian response, as reflected by estradiol and progesterone levels in serum
(figure 4). The mean estradiol and progesterone levels of the cycles induced with
15 - 20 µg/pulse were all above those obtained in cycles with 2.5 - 5 µg/pulse.
Both of them were higher than those observed in normal menstrual cycles
(Leyendecker et al., 1975). The results depicted in figure 4 were all obtained in
patients suffering from hypothalamic amenorrhea grade 3b.

Substitution during the Luteal Phase

The normal luteotrophic hormone in the human is pituitary LH (Van de Wiele et al.,
1970). In severe hypothalamic amenorrhea corpus luteum function immediately caeses
following termination of pulsatile Gn-RH substitution a few days after ovulation
(Leyendecker and Wildt, 1981). Continuation of pulsatile administration of Gn-RH
during the whole luteal phase resulted in normal luteal function as indicated by the
length of the luteal phase, the progesterone levels in serum and conceptions.
Previously, it was suggested to support the luteal function by one to three injections of 2500 IU of HCG once ovulation had been obtained by Gn-RH (Leyendecker
et al.,1980b) There is, however, no indication on the basis of our data
(Leyendecker and Wildt, 1983b) that one method of luteal substitution is superior
over the other in terms of pregnacy rate obtained.

Intravenous Versus Subcutaneous Application of Gn-RH

The same catheter used for the i.v. application of Gn-RH was also used for the
subcutaneous route, however without the addition of heparin to the hormone
containing solution. The catheter was placed into the fat tissue of the lower
abdominal wall. Ovulations could be induced with doses of 5 - 20 µg/pulse in
patients with hypothalamic amenorrhea of grades 2 - 3b and with 20 µg/pulse in a
patient with hypothalamic amenorrhea grade 3c following the removal of a cranio-
pharyngeoma (Leyendecker and Wildt, 1981). Four pregnancies were obtained with the
s.c. route. However, in contrast to the i.v. application with a 100% ovulation
rate, the adequate dose per pulse provided, there was an incidence of only 13
ovulatory cycles in 21 s.c. applications of Gn-RH. However, all these patients
who did not ovulate during s.c application, had ovulatory cycles when Gn-RH was
intravenously applied at the same dose level. Delayed resorption of Gn-RH from the
subcutaneous fat tissue might result in insufficient serum levels of Gn-RH for
adequate stimulation of the pituitary gonadotrophs.

Ovulation- and Pregnancy-Rate

The adequate dose of Gn-RH provided (15 - 20 µg/pulse i.v. in hypothalamic amenorrhea grade 3c and 2.5 - 5 µg/pulse in grades 3b - 2) ovulation and normal luteal
function can be expected in every treatment cycle. The ovulation rate is reduced,
when the s.c. route is chosen. Definitive treatment failure (no ovulation) was
only observed when the diagnosis of hypothalamic amenorrhea was not correct.
In the beginning of our studies, mild hyperandrogenemia was not taken into account
carefully. In these patients pulsatile administration of Gn-RH could not induce
ovulatory cycles. PCO and related pathological entities are, on the basis of our
experiencies, not considered to be suitable for pulsatile Gn-RH administration.
Recent studies indicate, however, that pulsatile Gn-RH treatment might be successfully applied in polycystic ovarian disease (Coelingh Bennink, 1983).

The pregnancy rate is remarkably high. Of 28 patients 24 became pregnant. One
patient had two successful pregnancies two years apart. Twenty one pregnancies
are completed with 26 children born, among them 3 sets of heterozygous twins and
one set of triplets. Five patients aborted of whom one patient had two sequential

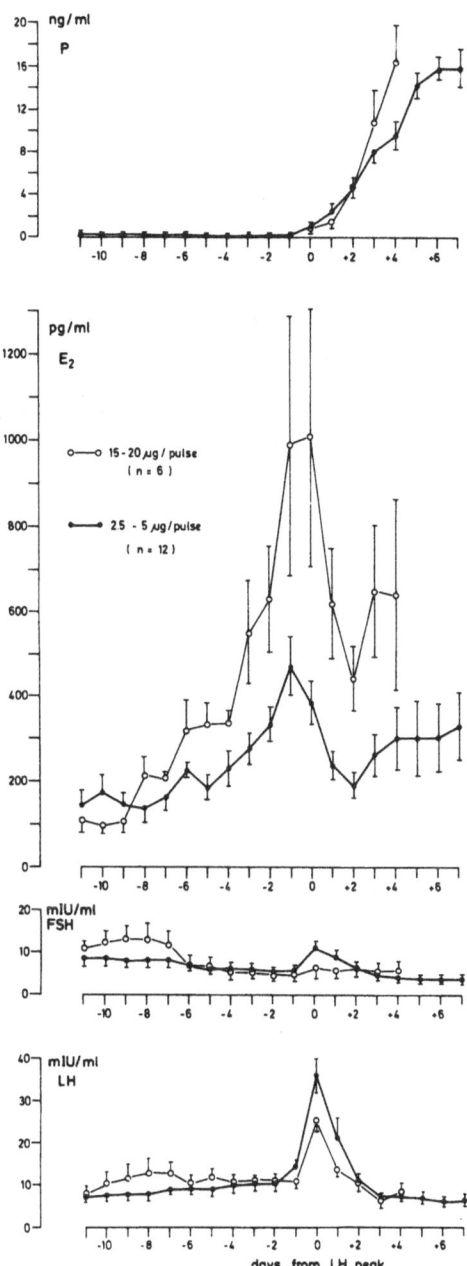

<u>Fig. 4.</u> The serum concentrations of FSH, LH, estradiol and progesterone in patients with hypothalamic amenorrhea grade 3b treated with 15 - 20 μg/pulse or with 2.5 - 5 μg/pulse of Gn-RH intravenously.

abortions probably due to active cytomegaly. Four of these patients conceived thereafter again and had uneventful pregnacies so far. Totally, 30 conceptions were
obtained in 28 patients.

The pregnancy rate, however, is critically dependent upon whether or not additional
factors causing infertility of the couple are present (i.e. tubal or andrological
factors). In "favourable couples", in whom the hypothalamic amenorrhea constitutes
the only cause of infertility of the couple, the pregnancy rate is comparable to that
of the normal population. Nineteen of 21 favourable couples achieved a pregnancy.
Ten conceptions occurred in the first, five in the second, three in the third and
one in the fourth treatment cycle. One patient, who had conceived in 1979 in her
first treatment cycle and had delivered a healthy girl in 1980, underwent another
treatment and conceived now in the fifth cycle. These data indicate a 60% chance
for favourable couples to achieve a pregnacy in the first treatment cycle.
Totally, 52 treatment cycles were applied in 21 favourable couples and 24 pregnancies were obtained (2.16 cycle per pregnancy).

In seven unfavourable couples only 5 pregnacies were achieved in 38 treatment
cycles. This poor result was mainly due to 2 patients with primary hypothalamic
amenorrhea, who conceived in their 6th and 9th cycle, respectively, following
insemination.

Ovarian Overstimulation and Multiple Pregnacies

The feedback mechanisms of ovarian steroids on the pituitary secretion of the
gonadotropic hormones are operative during pulsatile administration of Gn-RH.
Clinical signs of ovarian overstimulation have therefore not been observed
during 130 experimental and treatment cycles. As shown in figure 4, there is,
however, a dose response relationship between the dose of Gn-RH and the ovarian
response, which is mediated by adose related pituitary secretion of gonadotropins.
If it is taken into consideration that the selection of the dominant follicle
and the suppression of the other accompanying follicles is dependent to a certain
degree upon the gonadotropic stimulation, it has to be expected that a gonadotropic
stimulation of the ovaries resulting in discrete chemical overstimulation must
cause an increased incidence of multiple pregnacies as compared to the normal
population. In our study 4 multiple pregnacies were obtained out of 30 conceptions.
One of these multiple pregnancies was obtained by too high a dose for the respective
grade (20 µg/pulse in grade 3b of hypothalamic amenorrhea).

CONCLUSIONS

Pulsatile administration of Gn-RH by means of a portable pump ("Zyklomat") has
proven to be an efficient and practical method for the induction of ovulation
as a treatment of infertility in hypothalamic amenorrhea. The results obtained
with this method of treatment are critically dependent upon the correct selection
of patients as far as the diagnosis of hypothalamic amenorrhea is concerned.
Patients with hypothalamic amenorrhea, previously treated with human gonadotropins
are suitable for this mode of treatment. Further intensive studies have to demonstrate whether other anovulatory conditions, such as polycystic ovarian disease
and hyperprolactinemia (Leyendecker et al., 1980a), are also suitable for pulsatile
Gn-RH administartion.

In our study 30 conceptions were obtained in 28 patients. These favourable results are
obtained due to a rather physiological stimulation of the ovaries during chronic
intermittent (pulsatile) administration of Gn-RH. On the basis of operating negative
and positive feedback mechanisms of the ovarian steroids on the pituitary secretion of the gonadotropins during treatment, the follicle itself regulates the
required amount of gonadotropin stimulation. However, since there is a relationship

between the ³Gn-RH dose per pulse applied and the reaction of the pituitary-ovarian axis, the lowest efficient dose of Gn-RH in reliably inducing ovulatory cycles should be chosen.

ACKNOWLEDGEMENT

The skillful technical assistance of Miss Roswitha Klasen is gratefully acknowledged.

REFERENCES

Belchetz PE, Plant TM, Nakai Y, Keogh EJ, Knobil E (1978) Hypophyseal responses to continous and intermittent delivery of hypothalamic gonadotropin releasing hormone (Gn-RH). Science 202: 631

Bergquist C, Nillius SJ, Wide L (1979) Reduced gonadotropin secretion in postmenopausal women during treatment with a stimulatory LRH analogue. J Clin Endocrinol Metab 49:472

Boyar RM, Finkelstein J, Roffwarg H, Kapen S, Weitzman ED, Hellman L (1972) Synchronization of augmentd luteinizing hormone secretion with sleep during puberty. N Eng J Med 287:582

Boyar RM, Katz J, Finkelstein J, Kapen S, Weiner H, Weitzman ED, Hellman L (1974) Anorexia nervosa: Immaturity of the 24-hour luteinizing hormone secretion pattern. N Eng J Med 291:861

Carmel PW, Araki S, Ferin M (1976) Pituitary stalk portal blood collection in rhesus monkeys: Evidence for pulsatile release of gonadotropin releasing hormone (Gn -RH). Endocrinology 99:243

Coelingh-Bennink HJT (1983) Induction of ovulation by pulsatile intravenous administration of LHRH in polycystic ovarian disease. Presented at the Sixty-Fifth Annual Meeting of The Endocrine Society, San Antonio, Texas, 1983. Published by The Endocrine Society, in Proprams and Abstracts, p 81

Crowley jr WF, McArthur JW (1980) Simulation of the normal menstrual cycle in Kallmann's syndrome by pulsatile administration of luteinizing hormone -releasing hormone (LH-RH). J Clin Endocrinol Metab 51:173

Dericks-Tan JSE, Hammer E, Taubert HD (1977) The effect of D-Ser (TBU)^6-LH-RH-EA^{10} upon gonadotropin release in normally cyclic women. J Clin Endocrinol Metab 45:597

Dierschke DJ, Bhattacharya AN, Atkinson LE, Knobil E (1970) circhoral oscillations of plasma LH levels in the ovariectomized rhesus monkey. Endocrinology 87:850

Katz JL, Boyar RM, Roffwarg H, Hellman L, Weiner H (1977) LHRH responsiveness in anorexia nervosa: Intactness despite prepubertal circadian LH pattern. Psychosom Med 39:241

Katzorke T, Popping D, Ohe von der M, Tauber PF (1980) Clinical evaluation of the effects of a new long acting superactive luteinizing-releasing hormone (LH-RH) analog. D-Ser (TBU)^6-des Gly-10-Ethylamide-LH-RH, in women with secondary amenorrhea. Fertil Steril 33:35

Keogh EJ, Mallal SA, Giles PFH, Evans DV (1981) Ovulation induction with intermittent subcutaneous LH-RH. Lancet I, 147

Klinefelter jr HF, Albright F, Griswold G (1943) Experience with a quantitative test for normal or decreased amounts of follicle stimulating hormone in the uterus in endocrinological diagnosis. J Clin Endocrinol Metab 3:529

Knobil E (1980) The neuroendocrine control of the menstrual cycle. Recent Prog Hormone Res 36:53

Knobil E (1981) Patterns of hypophysiotropic signals and gonadotropin secretion in the rhesus monkey. Biol Reprod 24:44

Knobil E, Plant TM, Wildt L, Belchetz DE, Marshall G (1980) Control of the rhesus monkey menstrual cycle: permissive role of hypothalamic gonadotropin releasing (Gn-RH). Science 207:1371

Leyendecker G (1979) The pathophysiology of hypothalamic ovarian failure - diagnostic and therapeutic considerations. Eur J Obstet Gynec Reprod Biol 9:175

Leyendecker G, Hinckers K, Nocke W, Plötz EJ (1975) Hypophysäre Gonadotropine und ovarielle Steroide im Serum während des normalen menstruellen Zyklus und bei Corpus-luteum-Insuffizienz. Arch Gynec 218:47

Leyendecker G, Struve T, Plotz EJ (1980a) Induction of ovulation with chronic-inter-mittent (pulsatile) administration of LH-RH in women with hypothalamic and hyperprolactinemic amenorrhea. Arch Gynecol 229:117

Leyendecker G, Wildt L, Hansmann M (1980b) Pregnancies following chronic-intermittent (pulsatile) administration of Gn-RH by means of a portable pump ("Zyklomat") - a new approach to the treatment of infertility in hypothalamic amenorrhea. J Clin Endocrinol Metab. 51:1214

Leyendecker G, Wildt L, Plotz EJ (1981) Die hypothalamische Ovarialinsuffizienz. Gynäkologe 14:84

Leyendecker G, Wildt L (1981) Chronisch intermittierende Gabe von Gn-RH. Ein Beitrag zur Physiologie und Pathophysiologie der endokrinen Regulation des menstruellen Zyklus sowie ein neues Verfahren zur Ovulationsauslösung bei hypothalamischer Amenorrhoe. Therapiewoche 31:6711

Leyendecker G, Wildt L (1983a) Control of gonadotropin secretion in the human female In: Brenner RM, Phoenix CH, Norman L (eds) Neuroendocrine aspects of Reproduction. Academic Press, New York

Leyendecker G, Wildt L (1983b) Induction of ovulation with chronic-intermittent (pulsatile) administration of Gn-RH in women with hypothalamic amenorrhea J. Reprod Fertil (in press)

Nakai Y, Plant TM, Hess DL, Keogh EJ, Knobil E (1978) On the sites of the negative and positive feedback actions of estradiol in the control of gonadotropin secretion in the rhesus monkey. Endocrinology 102:1008

Nakano R, Washio M, Hashiba N, Tojo S (1982) Ovarian morphologic features and endocrine profile in amenorrhoic patients. Gynecol Obstet Invest 14:19

Santen RJ, Bardin CW (1973) Episodic luteinizing hormone secretion in man. Pulse analysis, clinical interpretation, physiologic mechanisms. J Clin Invest 52:2617

Schoemaker J, Simons AHM, Burger CW, Delemarred HA, van Kessel H (1982) Induction of ovulation with LH/FSH-releasing hormone (LH-RH) In: Rolland R, van Hall EV, Hillier SG, McNatty P, Schoemaker J (eds) Follicular Maturation and Ovulation. Excerpta Medica, Amsterdam and New York, p 373

Skarin G, Nillius SJ, Wide L (1982) Intermittent low dose luteinizing hormone - releasing hormone therapy for induction of normal ovulatory menstrual cycles in women with amenorrhea In: Rolland R, van Hall EV, Hillier SG, McNatty P, Schoemaker J (eds) Follicular Maturation and Ovulation. Excerpta Medica, Amsterdam and New York, p 398

Van de Wiele RL, Bogumil J, Dyrenfurth I, Ferin M, Jewelewicz R, Warren M, Rizkhallah T, Mikhail G (1970) Mechanisms regulating the menstrual cycle in women. Recent Progr Hormone Res 26:63

Van Vugt DA, Diefenbach WP, Ferin M (1983) Gonadotropin releasing hormone is detect-able in CSF collected from the third ventricle of monkeys and is distinctly pulsatile. Presented at the Sixty-Fifth Annual Meeting of The Endocrine Society, San Antonio, Texas, 1983. Published by The Endocrine Society, in Programs and Abstracts, p 126

Wildt L, Schwilden H, Wesner G, Roll, C, Brensing KA, Luckhaus J, Bähr M, Leyendecker G (1983) The pulsatile pattern of gonadotropin secretion and follicular develop-ment during the menstrual cycle and in women with hypothlamic and hyperandrogen-emic amenorrhea In: Leyendecker G, Stock H, Wildt L (eds) Brain and Pituitary Peptides II. Pulsatile administration of Gn-RH in hypothalamic failure: Basic and clinical aspects. Karger Verlag, Basel (in press)

Yen SSC, Tsai CC, Naftolin F, van den Berg G, Ajabar L (1972) Pulsatile pattern of gonadotropin release in subjects with and without ovarian function. J Clin Endocrinol Metab 34:671

Weitzman ED, Boyar RM, Kapen S, Hellman L (1975) The relationship of sleep and sleep stages to neuroendocrine secretion and biological rhythms in man. Rec Progr Hormone Res 31:399

Antigonadal Properties of LHRH Agonists: Therapeutical Applications in Human

M. Schmidt-Gollwitzer[1], W. Hardt[1], T. Genz[1], and V. Borgmann[2]

[1] Poliklinik und Frauenklinik des Klinikum Charlottenburg (Direktor Prof. Dr. G. Kindermann)
[2] Urologische Klinik des Klinikum Charlottenburg (Direktor Prof. Dr. R. Nagel)
  Freie Universität Berlin, D-1000 Berlin

INTRODUCTION

The hypothalamic pituitary system is responsible for proper gonadal function. Secretion of the gonadotropins is on the one hand maintained by the release at regular intervals of gonadotropin releasing hormone (pulsatile secretion of LHRH), and on the other hand positively or negatively modulated by the sexual steroids (Knobil 1980).

Unphysiologically high concentrations of LHRH are followed, after an initial stimulation phase due to a reduction in pituitary receptors, by both a decrease in gonadotropin secretion and dissociation of the LH/FSH ratio. This pathological mechanism can be accentuated by the biologically more effective LHRH agonist (Sandow et al. 1978). Repeated application leads to a secondary reduction of gonad function (Schmidt-Gollwitzer et al. 1979). This paradoxical antigonadal effect of LHRH agonist offers new prospects for fertility control and ablative endocrine therapy.

In this article, the results of our clinical experimental studies with the potent LHRH agonist Buserelin are summarized.

ANTIGONADAL EFFECT

Single dose application of the LHRH agonist Buserelin leads to a more prolonged and marked secretion of gonadotropins, compared with the effects of natural LHRH (Dericks-Tan et al. 1977). The pituitary reaction in sexually mature women is most vigourous at mid-cycle, maximal release occurring after an interval of 2 to 8 hours. Release of LH is substantially higher than that of FSH (Fig. 1a). Application over several days produces a marked decline in pituitary reaction, accompanied by almost complete suppression of FSH secretion (Fig. 1b).

Concomitant with the release of gonadotropins, single dose application of the LHRH agonist leads to stimulation and several days' application to reduction of sexual steroid production (Fig. 2). It is thus possible to exert a regulatory influence on the cyclic ovarian function. Intranasal (i.n.) application of the LHRH agonist provides a clinically acceptable method, in contrast to intravenous or subcutaneous application.

The LHRH agonist Buserelin was kindly supplied by
Dr. M. von der Ohe, Hoechst AG, Frankfurt a.M., Germany.

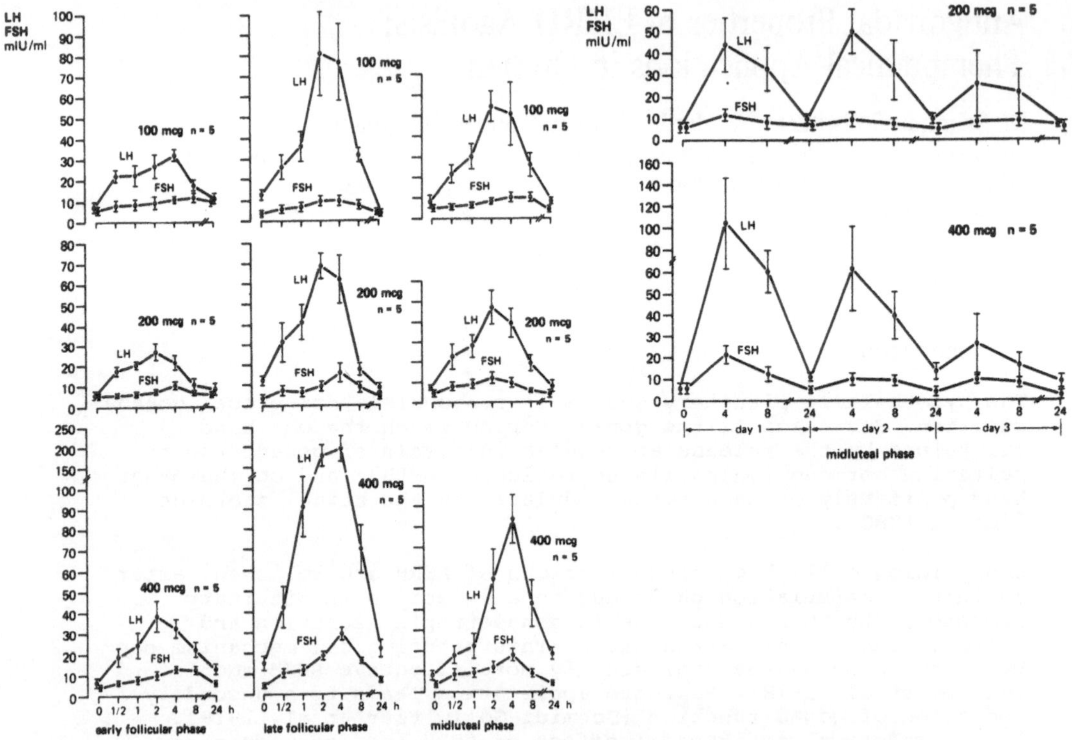

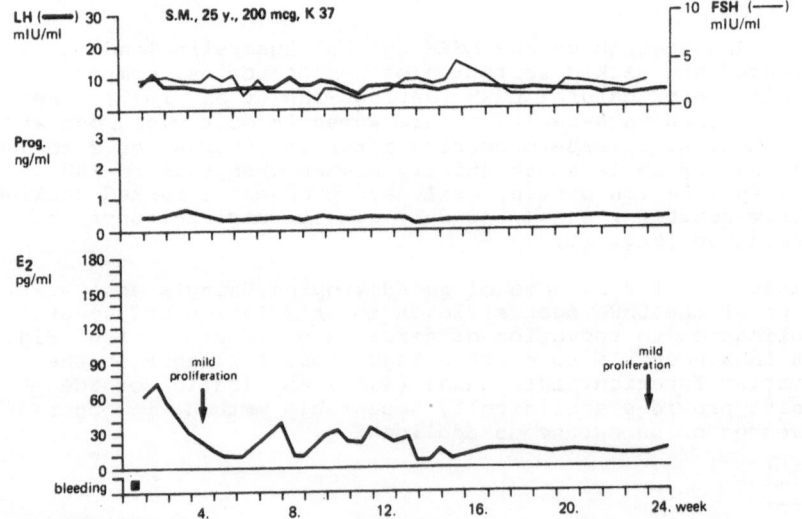

Fig. 1. Secretion profiles of gonadotropins during different phases of the menstrual cycle after intranasal application of different doses of Buserelin (a = single stimulation, b = stimulation over 3 days)

Fig. 2. Basal hormone profile during the course of daily treatment with Buserelin

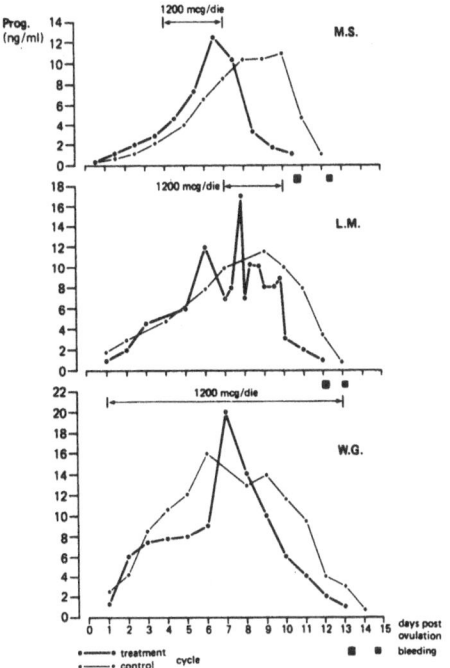

Fig. 3. Influence of i.n. Buserelin on corpus luteum function

Influencing various cyclic phases

Whereas luteolysis, leading to abortion, can be induced by the
LHRH agonists in animal experiments (rats, guinea-pigs, primates),
the results obtained with fertile women are by no means so straight
forward and promizing. Although the initial enhancement of
progesterone synthesis is succeeded by a post-stimulatory decline,
the progesterone levels remain within the range typical for normal
corpus luteum function (Fig. 3).

Even highly dosed subcutaneous application (100 % compared to 1-
2.5 % resorption after intranasal application) at various stages
of the luteal phase, failed to produce concrete evidence of a
sure luteolytic effect of the LHRH agonist in humans, either in
terms of the measured progesterone values or in terms of significant
shortening of the luteal phase (Fig. 4).

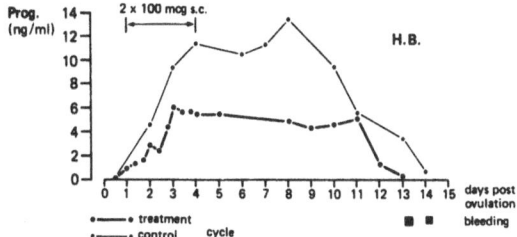

Fig. 4. Influence of s.c. Buserelin on corpus luteum function

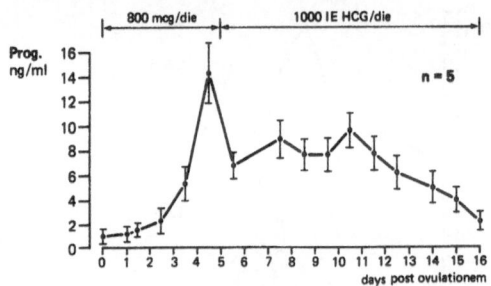

Fig. 5. Prolongation of corpus luteum function with human chorionic
gonadotropin after treatment with Buserelin (n = 5)

Furthermore, the reduction of progesterone synthesis induced by
the agonist can be reversed by human chorionic gonadotropin, and
the luteal phase prolonged beyond the normal duration (Fig. 5).
Even in cases where a pregnancy has occurred immediate reactivation
of the corpus luteum can be expected. Thus, the idea of post-
ovulatory contraception using LHRH agonists, put forward by Casper
et Yen (1979) and Lemay et al. (1980) is not a practicable approach.
Compared to the stable corpus luteum function, the more complex
process of follicle ripening appears to be more susceptible to
the influence of LHRH agonists. Follicle ripening can be disturbed
by the drug as a function of both time and dose.

Low doses (up to 200 mcg/day i.n.), starting at menstruation,
produce a fall in the estradiol level following an initial
stimulation. The treatment thus leads to delay of ovulation, which
in the low dose range depends on the duration of the application.
The succeeding corpus luteum function is not impaired (Fig. 6).

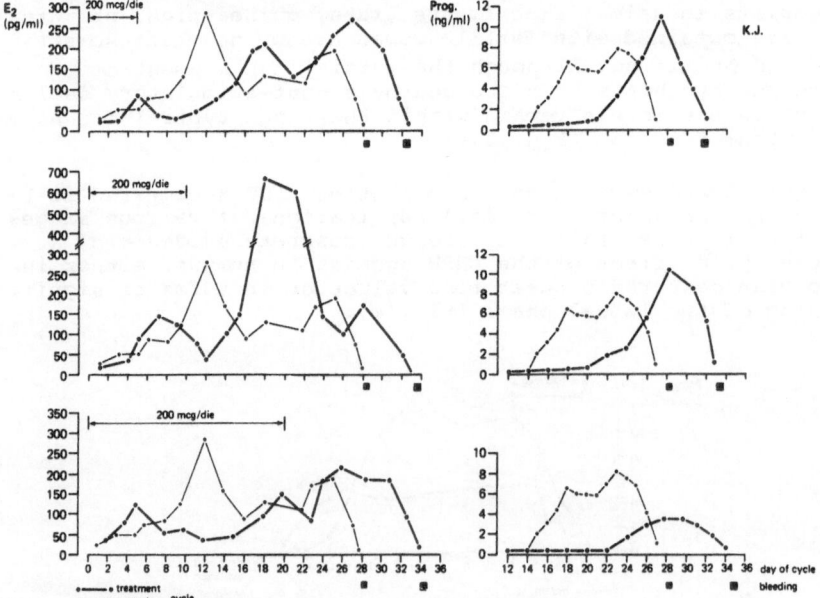

Fig. 6. Hormone profiles of sexual steroids during and after
treatment with Buserelin (200 mcg/d)

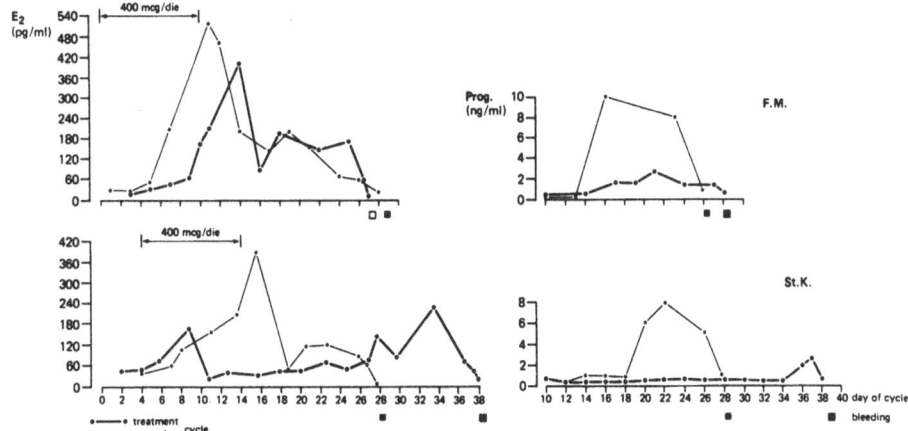

<u>Fig. 7.</u> Hormone profiles of sexual steroids during and after
treatment with Buserelin (400 mcg/d)

Higher doses (400 mcg/day i.n.), on the other hand, applied over
the same period, more frequently lead to impairment of the corpus
luteum function, and after 20-day application, to inhibition of
ovulation, which, however, is dependant on beginning treatment
early (Fig. 7). To obtain reproducible inhibition of ovulation,
medication must be commenced before the 5th day of cycle, otherwise
the process of selection of the dominant follicle can no longer
be interrupted with certainty. The inhibiting effect, particularly
after the 7th day, then becomes an ovulation inducing effect.

Delay or inhibtion of ovulation results in menstrual bleeding at
unpredictable times, showing that control of the cycle is no
longer possible. The short-term effect on follicle ripening as
a means of long-term fertility control is thus shown to be scarcely
practicable. The extent to which the proven inhibition of ovulation
can be maintained over longer periods, remained to be clarified.

Continuous Medication

Continuous treatment, as a function of dose, can be used to inhibit
ovulation over a period of months or years. With doses up to 200
mcg, progesterone values in as many as 85 % of the therapy months
were found indicative of either certain anovulation, luteinization
of non-ruptured follicles or severe corpus luteum insufficiency.
Increased dosage to 400 mcg daily produces this condition in 97
% of therapy months (Schmidt-Gollwitzer et al. 1981). For doses
above 400 mcg, anovulation can be shown in practically 100 % of
the medication medication months.

In contrast to the inhibition of ovulation, which is clearly dose
dependant, the effect on estrogen production, even at contraceptive
levels of the LHRH agonist, is very variable. Whereas in a number
of cases an abrupt restriction of estrogen secretion with consequent
amenorrhea at an early stage was found, the majority showed,
albeit with decreasing tendency, considerable variations in the
estradiol level up to levels of the preovulatory phase (Fig. 8).
This indicates that the effect on the follicle ripening mechanism
at contraceptive doses is individually very variable, with two
thirds of the women showing mainly irregular bleeding patterns,

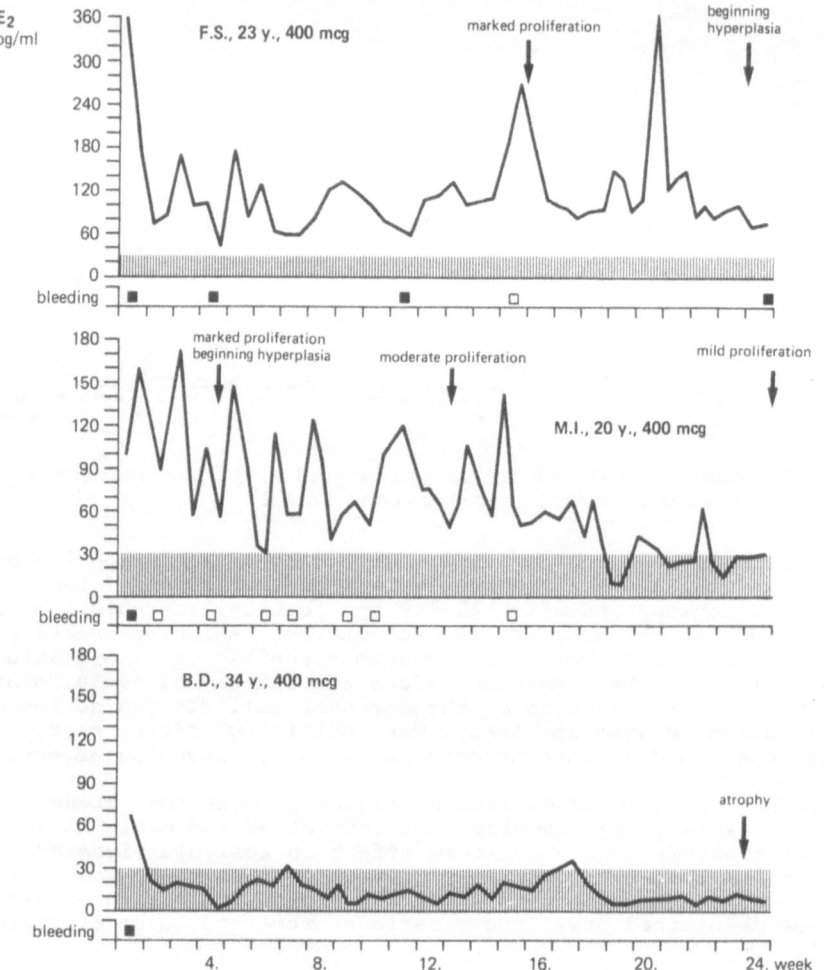

Fig. 8. Typical estradiol profiles during the continuous treatment with Buserelin

resulting from desynchronized endometrium formation. Endometrium biopsies repeated during different therapy months indicate both phases of prolonged and enhanced endometrium stimulation as well as phases of insufficient or non existent stimulation (inactivity or atrophy). Atypical endometrium hyperplasia was found in no cases. Declining estrogen secretion further resulted in a corresponding reversal of the initially present hyperplastic changes in the endometrium (Hardt et al.1981).

CLINICAL APPLICATION

The possibility of long-term fertility control and ablative endocrine therapy with LHRH agonists has been confirmed by our studies. Acceptance of the intranasal method of application was found to be very high. In addition, experimental findings confirm that this agonist has no measurable effect on essential metabolic functions - in contrast to the sexual steroids conventionally used for contraception.

Contraception

Continuous medication is, however, accompanied by loss of control
of menstrual bleeding. Since a decrease in estrogens down to pre-
or postmenopausal levels is generally to be expected in the course
of treatment, phases of uninhibited estrogen effects on the
endometrium, except in occasional cases, are unlikely, more
probable are the results of long-term estrogen deficiency. It
thus became desirable to develop a new treatment schedule which
guarantees the contraceptive as well as estrogenic effect on the
one hand, and permits better cycle control on the other.

Our approach was to determine to what extent cycle control could
be achieved by discontinuous medication (3 weeks treatment, one
weak's break). In view of the persistent disturbance of follicle
ripening by the above mentioned 20-day treatment, it was assumed
that intercurrent ovulation would hardly be likely during one
week's break. To ensure regular menstruation during the treatment
breaks, the discontinuous LHRH medication was combined with a
short-term gestagen therapy (20th-22nd day). The results of the
clinical tests with 21 volunteers over 101 months of treatment
show this approach to be feasible (Hardt et al. 1982).

At doses of 400 mcg, the contraceptive effect was maintained in
spite of the week's break. In contrast to the continuous treatment
(33 % regular bleeding) the discontinuous medication, with
additional gestagen therapy, produced a regular bleeding pattern
in the majority of women (4/5 of the volunteers, Fig. 9). In 1/5
of the group however, early ovarian suppression occurred in spite
of discontinuous treatment, resulting in intermittent bleeding,
with or without menstruation in the break, or amenorrhea (Fig.
10). Biopsies revealed that the degree of endometrium proliferation
was insuffizient to allow induction of menstruation by gestagen
treatment. In the majority of women, however, hormone levels and
biopsies before, during and after menstruation showed cyclic

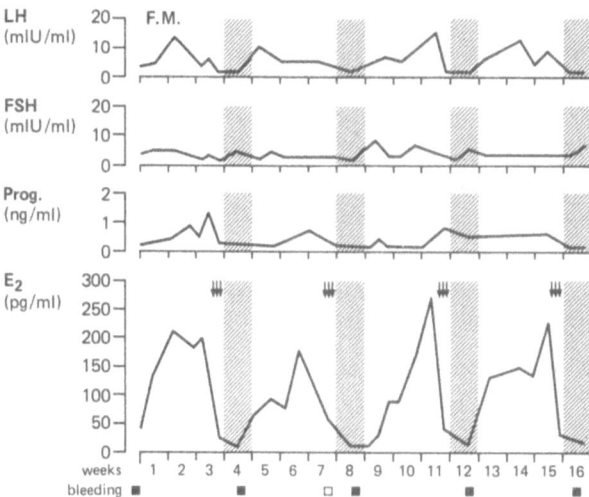

Fig. 9. Discontinuous treatment with 400 mcg Buserelin
(arrow = 10 mg norethisterone enanthate)

56

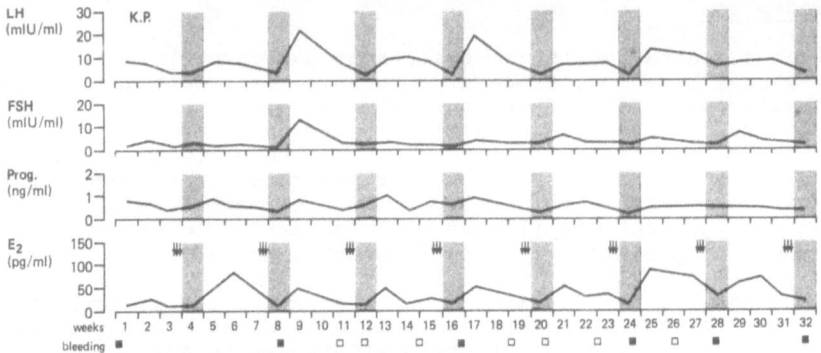

Fig. 10. Discontinuous treatment with 400 mcg Buserelin
(arrow = 10 mg norethisterone enanthate)

estrogen secretion as well as proliferation, transformation and
desquamation of the endometrium in accordance with the findings
expected during a normal cycle (Fig. 9).

Thus the risk of uninhibited estrogen influence on the endometrium
appears to be avoidable by combination of the LHRH treatment with
gestagen therapy which produces menstruation.

Discontinuous medication thus appears to represent a practicable
fertility control procedure. This is currently being tested for
its clinical usefulness in a multicentre study.

Ablative Endocrine Therapy

Ablative endocrine therapy in the cause of benign or malignant
hormone dependant disorders, can lead to an improvement in the
condition by interruption of the gonad function. The conventional
procedures as operative or radiogenic castration are definitive
and should only be carried out when the hormone sensitivity of
malignant disorders has been established with certainty. In order
to determine this dependance, as well as for the treatment of
benign conditions, such as endometriosis or precocious puberty,
reversible procedures for gonad suppression are desirable. High
doses of sexual steroids are only of limited acceptability in
view of their not inconsiderable side effects.

With high doses of the LHRH agonist Buserelin (800-1200 mcg/day),
intranasally administered, steroidogenesis in both men and women
can be suppressed for prolonged periods (Borgmann et al. 1982,
Hardt and Schmidt-Gollwitzer 1983). The measured testosterone or
estradiol values correspond to these found after surgical gonadectomy (Fig. 11).

The time required for complete pharmacological castration in women
is longer than that in men, or at least unpredictable within
certain limits (2-12 weeks). After termination of treatment, the
gonad function reverts to normal within a short time (2-8 weeks).

Our experinece so far with the LHRH agonist Buserelin is that the
suppression of testosterone secretion in men with metastasizing

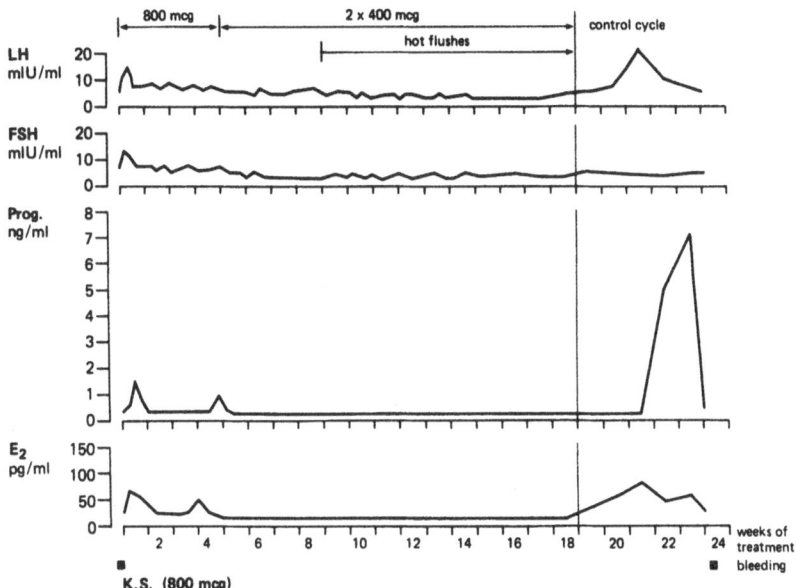

__Fig. 11.__ Reversible pharmacological castration with Buserelin

prostate carcinomas can be maintained as long as required. The
degree of remission achieved by this pharmacological castration
corresponds to that obtained by definitive surgical castration.
Above all, the possibility of testing the hormone dependance of
the tumor before performing irreversible surgical castration, as
well as the therapeutic possibilitiès of this psychologically
less distressing procedure, have substantially extended the scope
of treatment for this disorder.

Decisive advantages have been gained in the treatment of
endometriosis. It is now possible to suppress completely ovarian
steroidogenesis without any of the side effects normally associated
with use of the related sexual steroids. Even though operative
treatment provides the only final cure for endometriosis, a primary
conservative attempt at treatment with drugs is both desirable
and reasonable, particularly for younger women who wish to have
children. This reversible pharmacological castration, which we
have been able to demonstrate for the first time, is clearly
superior to other drug treatments so far available in view of the
high efficiency, reversibility and the absence of side effects,
and is expected to become the method of choice within the
foreseeable future.

SUMMARY

The development of the LHRH agonists have given rise to partly
unexpected therapeutical possibilities for influencing the gonad
function. They can be used for fertility control and for ablative
endocrine therapy of hormone dependant disorders. In view of its
specific pituitary point of attack, the rapid reversibility of

its effects and non-interference with metabolic processes, these drugs are likely to take an important place in the future as an interdisciplinary therapeutic tool.

REFERENCES

Borgmann V, Hardt W, Schmidt-Gollwitzer M, Adenauer H, and Nagel R (1982): Sustained suppression of testosterone production by the LH-RH agonist Buserelin in patients with advanced prostate carcinoma - A therapeutical approach. Lancet 1083:1097-1099

Casper RF, and Yen SCC (1979): Induction of luteolysis in the human with a long-acting analog of luteinizing hormone-releasing factor. Science 205:408-410

Dericks-Tan JSE, Hammer E, and Taubert H-D (1977): The effect of D-Ser(TBU)6-LH-RH-EA10 upon gonadotropin release in normally cyclic women. J Clin Endocrinol Metab 45:597-599

Hardt W, Schmidt-Gollwitzer M, von der Ohe M, and Nevinny- Stickel J (1981): Der Einfluß der Dauermedikation des LH-RH-Analogons Buserelin auf die Zyklusregulation. Geburtsh Frauenheilk 421:791-796

Hardt W, Schmidt-Gollwitzer K, Nevinny-Stickel J, and Schmidt-Gollwitzer M (1982): Fortschritte in der kontrazeptiven Anwendung des LH-RH-Agonisten Buserelin: Diskontinuierliche Medikation mit gestageninduzierter Abbruchblutung. Geburtsh Frauenheilk 42:874-877

Hardt W, and Schmidt-Gollwitzer M (1983): Sustained gonadal suppression in fertile women with the LHRH agonist buserelin. Clin Endocrinol 19:613-617

Knobil E (1980): The neuroendocrine control of the menstrual cycle. Recent Prog Horm Res 36: 53-88

Lemay A, Labrie F, Belanger A, and Raynaud J-P (1979): Luteolytic effect of intranasal administration of D-Ser (TBU)6, des-Gly-NH2-10 lueinizing hormone releasing hormone ethylamide in normal women. Fertil Steril 32:646-651

Sandow J, von Rechenberg W, Jerzabek G, and Stoll W (1978): Pituitary gonadotropin inhibition by a highly active analog of luteinizing hormone-releasing hormone. Fertil Steril 30:205-212

Schmidt-Gollwitzer K, Hardt W, Rebholz G, and Schmidt-Gollwitzer M (1979): The effect of a new longacting LH-RH analogue (HOE 766) on gonadotropin and steroid secretion in amenorrhoic women. Acta Endocrinol Suppl 225:357

Schmidt-Gollwitzer M, Hardt W, Schmidt-Gollwitzer K, and Nevinny-Stickel J (1981): Influence of the LH-RH analogue buserelin on cyclic ovarian function and on endometrium. Contraception 23:187-196

Structure-Function Relationships of Gonadotropins: Human Choriogonadotropin as a Model

W. E. Merz

Department of Biochemistry II, University of Heidelberg, Im Neuenheimer Feld 328, D-6900 Heidelberg

INTRODUCTION

Human choriogonadotropin (hCG) is a glycoprotein hormone which is synthesized by the syncytiotrophoblast (Midgley and Pierce 1962) of the placenta predominantly in the first trimester·of pregnancy. This hormone shows a close relationship to hypophyseal gonadotropins lutropin (LH) and follitropin (FSH) and to thyrotropin (TSH) concerning their amino acid sequences (Pierce and Parsons 1981). These glycoprotein hormones are composed of two dissimilar noncovalently linked subunits, α and β (Swaminathan and Bahl 197o; Canfield et al 1971). The α-subunit of hCG, molecular weight 14 9oo, consists of 92 amino acid residues (Bellisario et al. 1973). The two carbohydrate moieties are linked by N-glycosidic bonds to asparagine residues (Kessler et al. 1979a). The similarity between hCG-α- and human LH-α-subunit is striking: The primary structures are completely identical a deletion of 3 and an inversion of 2 residues excepted (Bellisario et al. 1973). In comparison to human LH and the other members of the superfamily, the β-subunit of hCG, molecular weight 23 ooo (Carlsen et al. 1973), shows 3o additional amino acids at the C-terminal region (residues 115-145) out of 145 residues (Birken and Canfield 1977; Keutmann and Williams 1977). In this region an hCG-specific antigenic determinant is located (Morgan et al. 1975; Talwar et al. 1976; Keutmann and Williams 1977; Matsuura et al. 1979; Ramakrishnan and Talwar 198o; Birken and Canfield 198o). Again homology between amino acid sequences of human LH and hCG in the common N-terminal peptide region is very distinct: Out of 115 amino acids 93 are identical (Birken and Canfield 198o). The molecule contains six carbohydrate moieties, 2 with N- and 4 with O-glycosidic linkages (Carlsen et al. 1973; Morgan et al. 1975; Birken and Canfield 198o). The structures of carbohydrate moieties of hCG are known (Kessler et al. 1979a,b). Marked differences exist between the carbohydrate compositions of hCG and LH (Papkoff and Li 197o; Sairam et al. 1974; Merz et al. 1974a; Kennedy and Chaplin 1976).

The homology in primary structures of LH and hCG is the basis for the complete cross-reaction in biological systems: Both hormones act via the same receptors and are identical in their ability to stimulate steroidogenesis mediated by activation of adenylate cyclase (Catt and Dufau 1978; Catt et al. 198o; Rommerts and Brinkman 1981). Pierce and coworkers (1971) demonstrated in an impressive experiment that hybrid molecules composed of e.g. LH-α and TSH-β subunits acted like that hormone from which β-subunit was taken. This clearly indicates, that receptor specificity seems to reside in the β-subunit portion. The function of the α-subunit is unknown and is the main issue of the following investigations. The α-subunits show higher homologies in their amino acid sequences. They might have more functions in common which are most essential since their primary structures are conserved to a high extent in evolution. Thus, investigations on the func-

tional role of the α-subunit of one of the hormones might provide information valid also for the others. The functional role of the α-
subunit might be:
1) To regulate biosynthesis and secretion of the hormone.
2) To induce a certain conformation of the β-subunit which results
   in organization of the receptor binding site.
3) To share in receptor binding together with the β-subunit.
4) To elicit hormone-induced metabolic activities in target cells
   subsequently to β-subunit mediated hormone receptor interactions.
In addition, Pierce and Parsons (1980) suggested other functions,
like protection of the hormone from rapid degradation and internalization of the α-subunit followed by induction of hormone-mediated metabolic events subsequently to receptor binding (in analogy to the
mode of action of some toxins like choleratoxin where the B-subunits
bind to GM1 receptors and the A-subunit portion is internalized and
then induces modulation of adenylate cyclase activity) (Dufau et al.
1978; Moss and Vaughan 1979).

The following investigations were performed in our laboratory in order to examine the particular role of the α-subunit for gonadotropic,
immunological, and physical properties of the hCG molecule as well as
for placental biosynthesis of this hormone.

RECOMBINATION OF SUBUNITS

The hormones of TSH-gonadotropin family can be dissociated into the
subunits by acidic pH conditions or urea (Swaminathan and Bahl 1970;
Aloj et al. 1973a; Morgan et al. 1974; Bewley et al. 1974; Ingham et
al. 1974). The isolated subunits seem to have no or only a very small
intrinsic biological activity (Catt et al. 1973; Morgan et al. 1974;
Merz et al. 1974b).
Recombination of the subunits completely restores the biological properties of the hormones (Aloj et al. 1973a; Ingham et al. 1976; Merz
1977; Strickland and Puett 1982). Our group showed for the first time
that recombination is accompanied by conformational changes and pas-
ses through definite transition states (Merz et al. 1973). Therefore,
study of recombination provides the key for understanding those molecular events which give rise to what we call organization of receptor
binding site. The time course of recombination measured with 3 methods
of different quality is shown in Fig. 1. HCG (Aloj et al. 1973a,b)-
like some other proteins (Brand et al. 1967; Jonas and Weber 1971;
Wildner 1976; Cody and Hazel 1977)-forms complexes with the fluorescence probe 1-anilinonaphthalene-8-sulfonate (ANS). The ligand is probably bound to hydrophobic domains of hCG. Intense protein-ligand interactions cause a 10-12 fold enhancement of ANS fluorescence when the
ligand is bound by the hormone. The isolated subunits lack this property (Aloj et al. 1973a,b). Thus, ANS fluorescence is used as a sensitive tool for measurement of recombination of native subunits (Aloj
et al. 1973a; Ingham et al. 1976; Merz 1977; Ingham and Bolotin 1978).
Restoration of immunological properties of hCG was measured by means
of an antiserum which specifically indicates antigenic determinants
which are expressed on native hCG but are missing on the isolated subunits. This antiserum was prepared by immunoabsorption of goat anti-
hCG antiserum with immobilized isolated hCG-subunits. In radioimmunoassay hCG/β-subunit cross-reaction of this purified antiserum
is smaller than 0.2%. After immobilization of this antiserum on Se-
pharose 4 B, binding of hCG recombined from ^{125}I-labelled α- + native β-subunit was measured (Merz, Hengen, Vörg, Dörner in preparation).
Biological activity in vivo was determined by means of rat prostate
assay which measures weight increase of accessory reproductive organs

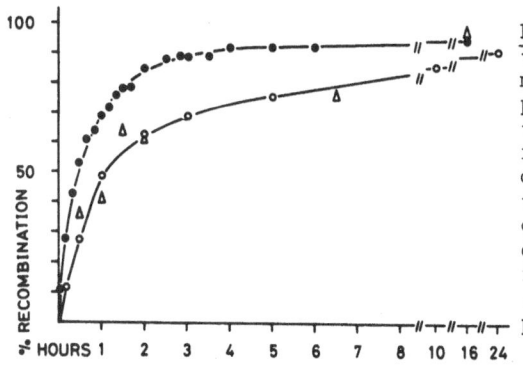

Fig. 1. Time course of recombination of isolated subunits of hCG
measured by means of selected properties of hCG, of which the isolated subunits are deficient. Fluorescence of hCG/ANS complexes (●),
quaternary structure specific antigenic determinant (○), and biological activity in vivo (▲). Protein
concentration at t=0 was 50 μM; buffer system as described elsewhere
(Merz et al. 1973) with addition of
penicillin G and streptomycin; 37°C.

caused by testosterone synthesized in Leydig cells which are the target cells for LH and hCG in the male. It is obvious that the ability
of hCG to enhance ANS fluorescence on the one hand and organization
of quaternary structure specific antigenic determinants and biological activity in vivo on the other hand follow different kinetics. We
conclude from these results that recombination proceeds at least in a
two step mechanism first leading to a physical association of the
subunits α + β ⇌ α · β, which does not result in a complete restoration of the properties of the hormone, followed by a slower process
of intramolecular reorientation, α · β ⟶ H, which completely
restores the properties of the native hormone. A two step model of
association of the subunits had been also described by others (Bewley
et al. 1974; Ingham et al. 1976). Bewley showed that recombination of
ovine LH subunits seems to proceed more rapidly when monitored by the
increase in sedimentation coefficient than by CD (circular dichroism).
These data excellently correlate with those presented in Fig. 1. In
contrary, Strickland and Puett (1982) could not find any indication
of existence of an intermediate.

MODIFICATIONS BY EXO- AND ENDOPROTEASES

Digestion with Carboxypeptidases

Carboxypeptidase A (EC 3.4.17.1) readily splits off residues 88 - 92
of the isolated α-subunit. The enzyme is stopped at Cys 87 which is
linked to Cys 59 by a disulfide bridge. Thus, a definite final product is yielded. Serine carboxypeptidase (EC 3.4.16.1) also releases
amino acids from the C-terminus of the isolated α-subunit much more
slowly, however. C-terminus of isolated native β-subunit is resistant
even against prolonged proteolytic attack by carboxypeptidase A whereas serine carboxypeptidase at pH 6.5 splits óff C-terminal residues
143-145. Carboxytermini of the subunits seem to be resistant to a
great extent when native hCG is digested by carboxypeptidase A. Serine
carboxypeptidase again releases the 3 residues from the C-terminus of
β-subunit. Recombination of des-(88-92)-α-subunit with native β-subunit is not affected by the modification yielding a single association
product when estimated by means of thin - layer gel filtration, ultracentrifugation, and immunological methods. The recombination products
containing an α-subunit portion with shortened C-terminus are biologically less active or even inactive in spite of presence of native
receptor-specific β-subunit in the modified hormone molecule. Impairment of biological functions of these recombination products extends
from receptor binding, hCG-induced stimulation of adenylate cyclase of

Table 1. Biological activity of choriogonadotropin with shortened C-terminus of α-subunit portion determined in three different bioassay systems.

No[a] Modified cho- riogonadotro- pin	Mol amino acids re- leased/mol protein	Residual activity[b,c] (95% Confidence limits)		
		Radioligand- receptor- assay[d] %	Stimula- tion of adenylate cyclase %	Rat pro- state assay %
1 des-Ser^{92}-α- + native β-subunit	Ser(.5)	60.4 (56.4-67.9)	52.6 (38.4-91.7)	48.2 (18.7-66.7)
2 des-Lys^{91},Ser^{92}-α- + native β-subunit	Lys(.6) Ser(1)	31.1 (23.1-35.3)	48.3 (42.3-77.7)	not deter- mined
3 des-(90-92)-α- + native β-subunit	His(.3)Lys(1) Ser(1)	32.1 (30.2-34.2)	44.3 (34.4-93.5)	40.0 (32.0-52.8)
4 des-(88-92)-α- + native β-subunit	Tyr(2)His(1) Lys(1)Ser(1)	1.2 (0.5- 1.9)	1.0 (0.5- 1.6)	0.0[f]

[a]α-subunit digested with carboxypeptidase A(No.1,2,4) or serine carboxypeptidase (No.3).
[b]Residual activity = 100 x activity modified hCG/activity native α- + native β-subunit.
[c]Recombination product of native subunits reached 9000-11000 IU/mg (=75-92% of hCG activity).
[d]Rat testes homogenate; ^{125}I-labelled hCG.
[e]Rat Leydig cells purified by Percoll density gradient centrifugation.
[f]No significant effect up to a dose of 1000 ng/animal.
Data were calculated from Merz (1979), Merz and Dörner (1979) and Merz and Sessler (1981).

rat Leydig cells to more indirect hormonal effects like stimulation of growth of accessory reproductive organs (Table 1) and regulation of testicular cytochrome P 450 content (Merz, Kühn-Velten, Sessler, Dörner in preparation).
The following questions arise:
Is the diminution of receptor binding ability and biological activi- ty caused by an impairment of those subunit interactions which organi- ze the binding sites on the receptor-specific β-subunit, or did the modification destroy receptor binding sites on the α-subunit? In the first case the modified recombined hormone should have a conformation discernable from native hCG. The competence for receptor specificity and binding may reside in β-subunit. In the second model, receptor- binding and receptor specificity is partitioned between α- and β-sub- unit. Thus, reaction mechanism of specific binding to receptor would be much more complicated than in the first case. Both theories are held in literature: Parson and Pierce (1979) failed to find a changed conformation by means of measurements of CD of recombination products of native bovine LH β-subunit and bovine LH α-subunit with a C-ter- minus shortened by five amino acid residues. In addition, they cross- linked the subunits in order to prevent their dissociation in biologi- cal test systems. In our experiments, we found marked differences in CD spectra of des-(88-92)-hCG-α-subunit and native α-subunit. CD spec-

tra of recombination products from native α- + native β-subunit and des-(88-92)-α- + native β-subunit, however, were identical (Merz 1979). This, of course, does not exclude existence of small conformational changes. As pointed out below immunological and physical investigations clearly indicate that small conformational changes, must have occurred:
1. Stepwise removal of amino acids from the C-terminus of the α-subunit gradually lowers quantum yield of fluorescence of ANS complex with modified hCG (Table 2). This is not caused by a loss of binding sites for ANS on the protein molecule which is evident from the fact that ANS-induced aggregation of hCG (Ingham et al. 1975) is observed both, with native and modified hCG. Especially no heterogeneity was observed, as far as can be concluded from thin-layer gel filtration experiments: The entire material seems to be aggregated in presence of ANS. This was confirmed by analytical ultracentrifugation experiments (Merz, Riesner in preparation). Modified hCG shows sedimentation in a single band in presence or in absence of ANS. ANS and protein moving boundaries migrate in the same band again indicating the ability of the modified hormone to bind ANS molecules. Thus, the

Table 2. Influence of enzymatic modification of hCG and isolated subunits by carboxypeptidases on the fluorescence of a complex of the hormone and 1-anilinonaphthalene-8-sulfonate (ANS).

Fluorescence at 489 nm (excitation at 38o nm) of protein solutions (5o or 1oo μM) in 2o μM ANS (magnesium salt) determined on ANS base line of fluorescence spectra.

No.[a]	Protein	Mol amino acids released/ mol protein	Relative ANS/hCG fluorescence ± SD	n
1	native hCG	-	1oo	
2	des-Ser^{92}-hCG	Ser(o.4)	56.0 ± 8.5	1o
3	des-(143-145)-hCG	Leu(1)Pro(1)Gln(1)	88.7 ± 5.o	5
4	native α- + native β-subunit	-	1oo	
5	native α- + des-Gln^{145}-β-subunit	Gln(o.3)	93.1 ± 2.3	6
6	native α- + des-(143-145)-β-subunit	Leu(1)Pro(1)Gln(1)	76.9	3
7	des-Ser^{92}-α- + native β-subunit	Ser(o.5)	5o.8 ± 6.3	8
8	des-Lys^{91},Ser^{92}-α- + native β-subunit	Lys(o.6)Ser(1)	36.3 ± 1.3	6
9	des-(88-92)-α- + native β-subunit	Tyr(2)His(1) Lys(1)Ser(1)	26.4 ± 2.3	1o

[a]Digestion with carboxypeptidase A(No. 2, 7-9) and serine carboxypeptidase (No. 3,5,6), respectively. Data taken from Merz (1979) and Merz and Dörner (1979).

diminished quantum yield of fluorescence is caused by a weakening of
binder-ligand interactions most probably due to small conformational
changes of hormone. The use of ANS as a reporter group for detection
of small conformational changes has been described also by others. In
some cases it seems to be more sensitive than CD measurements (Cheung
and Morales 1969; Müller 1979; Yoshinaga 1976; Wildner 1976).
2. Additional support for the presence of conformational changes in
the recombination product des-(88-92)-α- + native β-subunit is deduced from immunological investigations. As it was shown above our purified hCG antiserum indicates antigenic determinants which seem to
be restored in the course of recombination in the second step during
conversion of α·β complex into the hormone. This antigenic determinant
depends on a certain conformation of hCG polypeptide chains. It is expressed only in the native hormone but does not seem to be expressed
in the modified recombination product (Fig. 2).

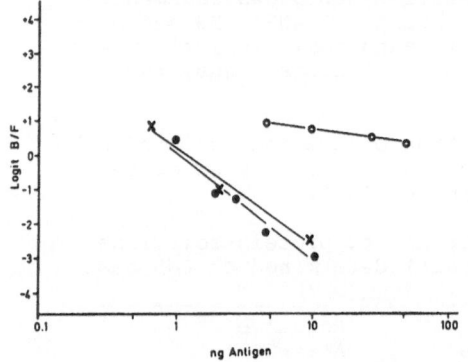

Fig. 2. Exemplification by
radioimmunoassay of a quaternary antigenic determinant in
native hCG (●) or hCG recombined from native subunits (X)
and absence of this structural
element in recombination product des-(88-92)-α- + native
β-subunit (O). Purified goat
antiserum against hCG and
125I-labelled hCG as trace was
used.

In conclusion, the significance of the C-terminal region of hCG-α-
subunit seems to be the following:
1. Structural integrity of the α-subunit is an essential precondition
for expression of biological activity of hCG.
2. A modification of the C-terminal region results in small conformational changes which prevent the subunits from interacting effectively.
3. Physical and immunological experiments have shown that the recombination product des-(88-92)-α- + native β-subunit differs in conformation from native hCG as well as from the hormone recombined from the
native subunits.
4. The receptor binding site which is supposed to be localized on the
β-subunit is incompletely organized if the α-subunit does not contribute to effective protein-protein interactions.

Digestion with Chymotrypsin and Trypsin

In the following some results obtained by digestion of the isolated α-
subunit and native hCG by endoproteases will be discussed. Digestion
of the isolated native hCG-α-subunit with chymotrypsin results in release of the heptapeptide, residues 41-47 and in cleavage of the peptide bond between phenylalanine residues 18 and 19 (Fig. 3). The methio-
nine-glycine bond (residues 29,3o) is also cleaved, however, at a very
slow rate. CD spectrum of the α-subunit digested by chymotrypsin is
significantly changed thus clearly indicating disturbance of the native
conformation of the α-subunit (Fig. 4). Recombination of the α-subunit
digested by chymotrypsin and the native β-subunit is not affected.
Fluorescence of a complex of the recombination product and ANS is reduced by 75 %. Biological activity in vivo (rat prostate assay) as well
as activity to stimulate rat Leydig cell adenylate cyclase is smaller

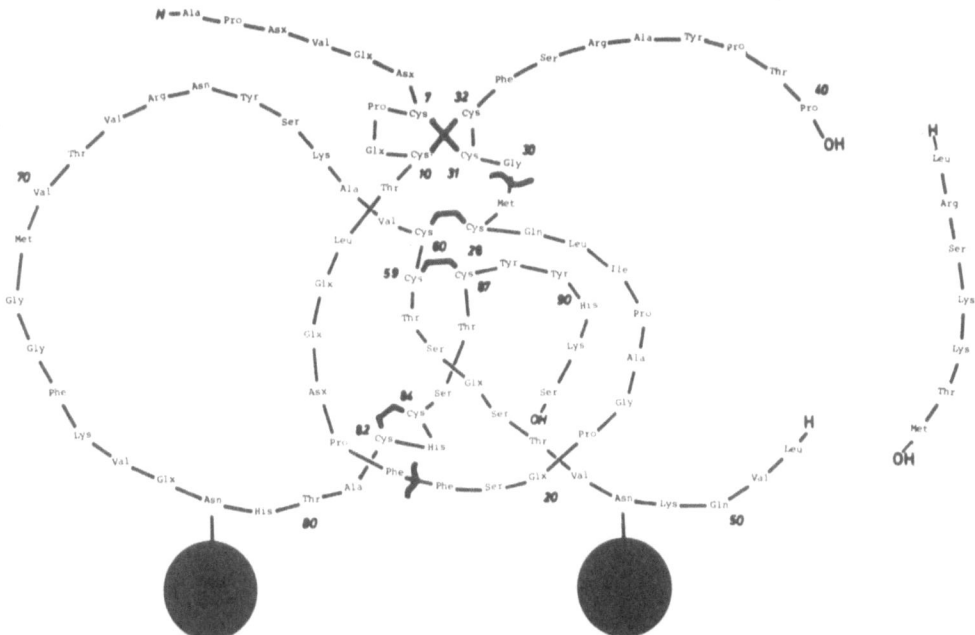

Fig. 3. Cleavage of isolated hCG-α-subunit by TLCK-treated chymotrypsin (2 h, 37°C, hCG: Chymotrypsin = 50:1 w/w). Arrangement of disulfide bridges (drawn in bold) according to Mise and Bahl (1980). Localization of cleavage positions by determination of N-termini of peptides separated by ion exchange chromatography and by gel filtration, and fingerprint and amino acid analysis; carbohydrate chains are attached to Asn residues 52 and 78.

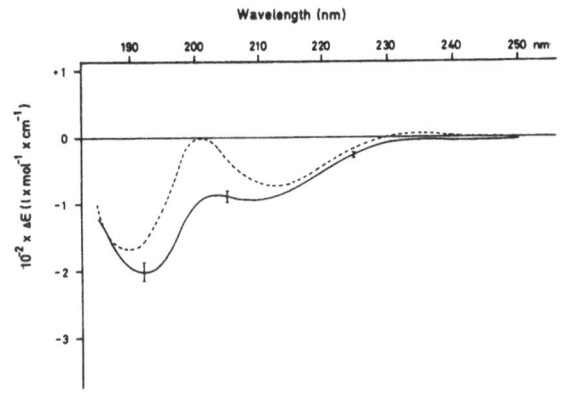

Fig. 4. Spectrum of circular dichroism of native hCG-α-subunit (——) and α-subunit digested by chymotrypsin (– – –). Protein concentration 1 mg/ml; 0.1 M phosphate buffer pH 7.5; 20°C. Vertical bars represent oscillation range of CD signal.

than 1 % in comparison to native hCG. Thus, a remarkable parallelism can be observed between these results and biological and physical properties of recombination products containing the native β-subunit and an α-subunit with shortened C-terminus. In the α-subunit digested by chymotrypsin the C-terminal region is still intact. Nevertheless, both digestions of the α-subunit by chymotrypsin as well as by carboxypeptidase A result in the same effect on biological activity and on hCG/ANS fluorescence of modified hormone although different regions of the

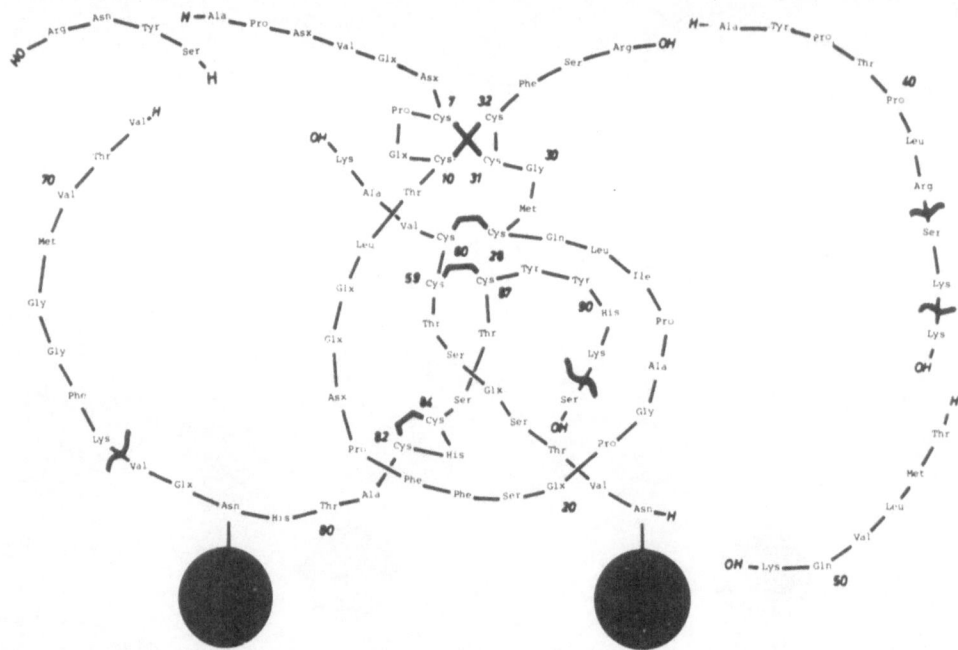

Fig. 5. Cleavage of isolated hCG-α-subunit by TPCK-treated trypsin
(2 h, 37°C hCG: trypsin = 50:1 w/w). Arrangement of disulfide bridges
(drawn in bold) according to Mise and Bahl (198o). Localization of
cleavage positions by determination of N-termini of the isolated peptides and by fingerprint and amino acid analysis. Carbohydrate chains
are attached to Asn residues 52 and 78.

α-subunit are affected. This seems to indicate that C-terminal region 88 - 92 of α-subunit is not directly involved in receptor
binding. In both cases, however, irreversible conformational changes
of the α-subunit seem to account for the loss of restoration of biological activity of recombination products. It is of interest that
native hCG is almost completely resistant to digestion by chymotrypsin.
Digestion of the native isolated α-subunit with trypsin within a few
minutes leads to cleavage of several peptide bonds (Fig. 5). The re-
mainder is a peptide designated α-T1. It contains the two carbohydrate chains and amino acid residues 1-35, 52-63 and 68-91 held together
by the 5 disulfide bridges of α-subunit. The peptide bonds Lys-Val
(residues 75,76) is not hydrolyzed unless incubation time is extended to 24 h. The α-T1 peptide core does not recombine with the native β-subunit. It is of interest that α-T1 peptide retains ordered
structural elements which is evident from CD-spectrum (not shown).
Immunological studies confirm this by the use of an antiserum against
native hCG-α-subunit which recognizes determinants of the isolated
subunit depending upon its intact conformation (Fig. 6). Peptide
α-T1 shows immunological properties more similar to native α-subunit
than the entire polypeptide chain of α-subunit after reduction of
disulfide bridges and alkylation of thiol groups. When native hCG is
digested by trypsin, the α-subunit remains remarkably stable, indicating that the cleavage positions are well protected in contrast to
isolated α-subunit (Fig. 7) (Merz, Merkel in preparation). The Arg-Phe
bond (residues 114,115) of the β-subunit seems to be hydrolyzed rapi-

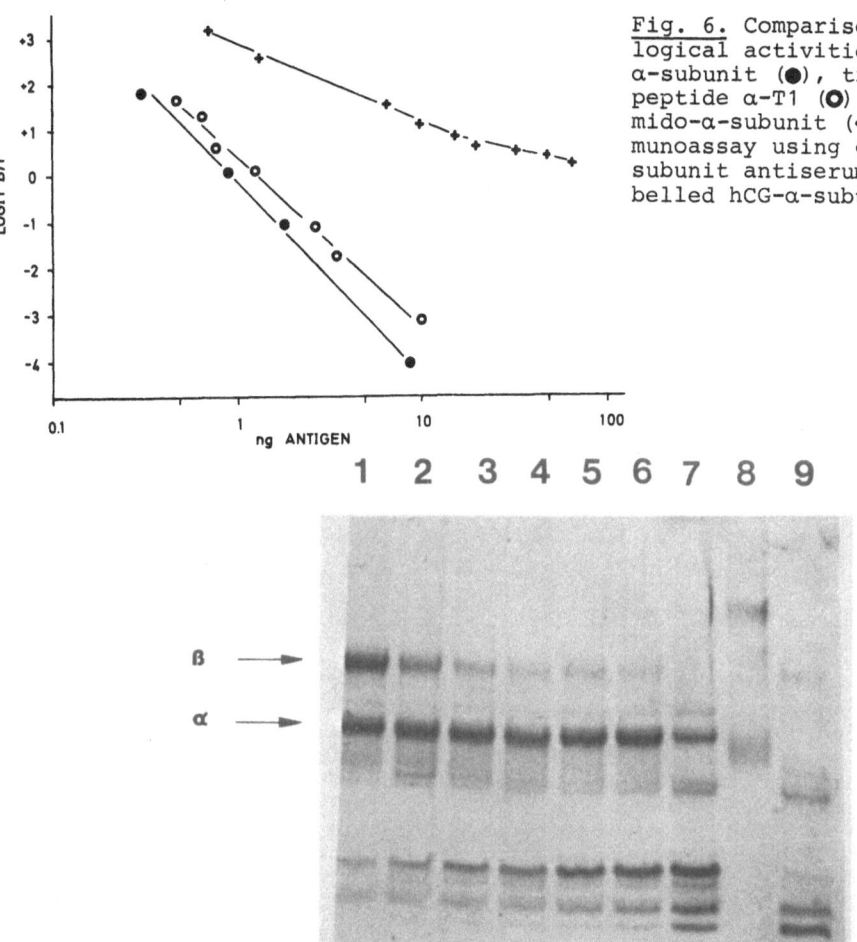

Fig. 6. Comparison of immunological activities of native
α-subunit (●), tryptic core
peptide α-T1 (O) and S-aceta-
mido-α-subunit (✦) in radioimmunoassay using goat anti α-
subunit antiserum and ^{125}I-la-
belled hCG-α-subunit as trace.

Fig. 7. Time course of digestion of native hCG by TPCK-treated trypsin
(Trypsin:hCG=1:2oo w/w; 37°C). SDS polyacrylamide gradient gel electrophoresis (Weber and Osborn 1969) (T:12-25%, C:2,5%). Aliquots taken from
hCG/trypsin incubation at intervals of 1o Min (lane 1=1o Min lane 6=
6o Min), and at 18o Min (lanes 7,8) and 22 h (lane 9). Incubation (2 Min,
Min, 95°C) prior to electrophoresis with SDS (O.7%)(lanes 1-9) and β-
mercaptoethanol (6.7%)(except lane 8).

dly. By this, however, the hCG-specific immunological domain is no
longer covalently attached to the molecule. This should be kept in
mind when using hCG as a tumor marker. Tumors very often activate or
secrete a variety of proteases which help the tumor to invade the sur-
rounding tissue. This may result in hormone fragments which show a
poor cross-reaction with antibodies directed against the native molecule as shown in Fig. 8 with one of our anti-hCG antisera. Birken and
Canfield (198o) have described cleavage of Arg-Phe bond (residues 114,
115) only in the case of the isolated β-subunit. The physiological re-
levance of the fact that this bond is also cleaved in native hCG as
described above seems to be evident from the occurrence of the C-terminal fragment hCG-β115-145 in urine of a woman with choriocarcinoma
(Amr et al. 1983).

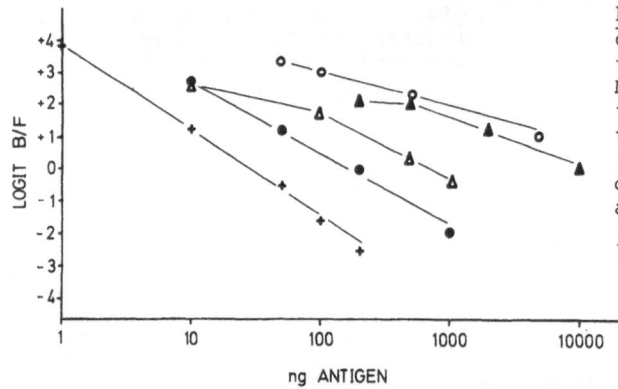

Fig. 8. Influence of digestion of native hCG by immobilized trypsin (Enzygel, Boehringer, Mannheim) on immunological activity in radioimmunoassay. Native hCG (✦), isolated α-subunit (△), isolated β-subunit (▲), digested hCG (●) (22 h, 37°C), and peptide fragment β 115-145 (⊙). Goat anti-hCG antiserum, ^{125}I-labelled hCG as trace.

CHEMICAL MODIFICATIONS

Modification by 1-Anilino-4-azidonaphthalene-8-sulfonate

Localization of ANS binding sites is of great interest for several reasons: Using a variety of different methods to modify the native hormone chemically or enzymatically we have found in many cases that the ability of a modified hormone to enhance ANS fluorescence corresponds to its biological activity. Furthermore, ANS is a sensitive probe to indicate small conformational changes. Therefore, a study of spatial relationship between receptor binding sites on one hand and ANS binding sites on the other is a point of great interest. For this reason we were the first to synthesize a 4-azido derivative of ANS in order to be able to perform photocoupling experiments (Böhm, Merz in preparation) (Fig. 9). The biological activity in vivo does not seem to be affected by ANS if one or two molecules are covalently linked to one molecule of hCG (Table 3). This indicates that the binding sites of the ligand are not identical with the biological active site of hCG. The binding sites for ANS and 4-azido-ANS seem to be identical as can be concluded from the fact that the binding of ANS is prevented by previous photocoupling of 4-azido-ANS. At present we are investigating the localization of 4-azido-ANS coupling sites on the subunits.

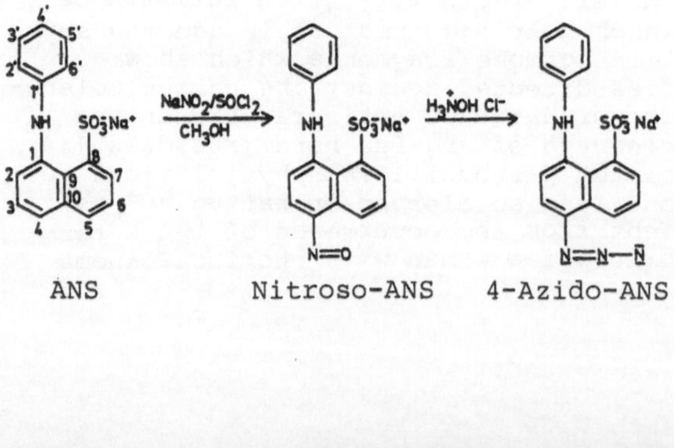

ANS   Nitroso-ANS   4-Azido-ANS

Fig. 9. Synthesis of 1-anilino-4-azidonaphthalene-8-sulfonate (4-azido-ANS) starting with N-nitrosation of ANS and conversion of nitroso-ANS with hydroxylammonia chloride to the azido derivative.

Table 3. Biological activity of hCG modified by photolytic coupling of 1-anilino-4-azidonaphthalene-8-sulfonate (4-azido-ANS).

Purified hCG (0.13-0.91 µmol) incubated for 30 Min at 0°C (pH 8.5) with indicated amount of 4-azido-ANS in the dark. Separation of excess of ligand by chromatography on Sephadex G25 column(1x30 cm). Photolysis induced by irradiation with mineral light (Camac TL-900) at wavelength 350 nm. Reaction products removed by gel filtration (Sephadex G25 column, 1x90 cm). Biological activity determined by rat prostate test, 2nd. Intern. Standard for Choriogonadotropin as reference substance.

Protein	Mol 4-azido-ANS /mol protein		Biological Activity		Precision
	Added	Incor-porated	IU/mg	95% Confidence limits	λ
native hCG	-	-	12 8oo	1o ooo - 17 2oo	o.192
hCG-(ANS)$_1$	1.5	1	11 4oo	9 1oo - 14 1oo	o.171
hCG-(ANS)$_2$	2.5	1.9	11 4oo	8 8oo - 15 6oo	o.199
hCG-(ANS)$_6$	8	5.6	8 5oo	6 6oo - 11 1oo	o.191

Iodination

HCG radioactively labelled with isotope ^{125}I is used for several purposes, e.g. radioimmunoassay (Vaitukaitis et al. 1971; Franchimont et al. 1971; Vaitukaitis et al. 1976), radioligand receptor assay (Catt et al. 1972; Leidenberger and Reichert 1972a; Saxena et al. 1974; Catt et al. 1976; Saxena 1976), and investigations on the internalization of the hormone by target cells (Leidenberger and Reichert 1972b; Amsterdam et al. 1979; Amsterdam et al. 1981; Ascoli 1981). It is a necessary precondition for these kinds of application that the labelled and the native hormone are completely identical. Investigation of this precondition is not easy since e.g. for physical studies higher concentrations are to be applied which will result in a mutual damage of the molecules by radioactive decay of the label. For these reasons, we have studied the influence of iodination on hCG by nonradioactive modification of the hormone. Nonradioactively iodinated hCG was prepared under mild conditions (molar ratio Chloramin T: iodine= 2.5:1) and in an amount of several milligrammes in order obtain sufficient material for preparative isolation. This allows a number of physical studies like spectroscopy which are impossible to perform with radioactive material. In addition, the activities of native and iodinated hCG can be directly correlated in competitive isotopic dilution assays. Incorporation of iodine was determined from the shoulder in ultraviolet spectrum at 3o5 nm which is the absorption band of phenolic hydroxyl group of tyrosine residues (Fig. 1o). When hCG is labelled with one atom of ^{125}I and dissociated into the subunits more than 90% of radioactivity comigrates with α-subunit band in SDS-polyacrylamide gel electrophoresis (Fig. 11). If the band is digested extensively by carboxypeptidase A, 8o% of the radioactivity is released from the α-subunit band. This indicates that tyrosines 88 and/or 89 are labelled by monoiodination mainly forming 3-iodo-tyrosyl residues. Biological activity in vivo of nonradioactive monoiodo-hCG is only slightly diminished but not significantly (based on 95% confidence limits (Table 4). Pentaiodo-hCG shows a significant lowering of biological activity in rat prostate assay. Receptor binding activity of mono-

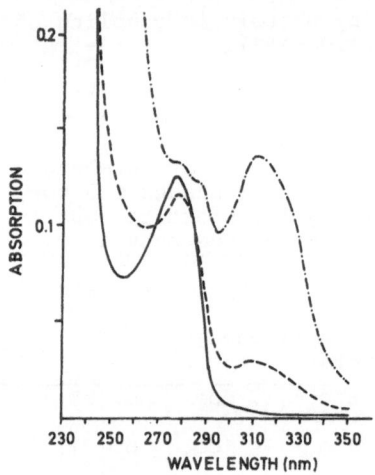

Fig. 1o. Ultraviolet spectra of native hCG (────), monoiodo-hCG (──-──), and pentaiodo-hCG (──·──).
O.2 M TRIS buffer pH 8.45, protein concentration 11,4 µM.

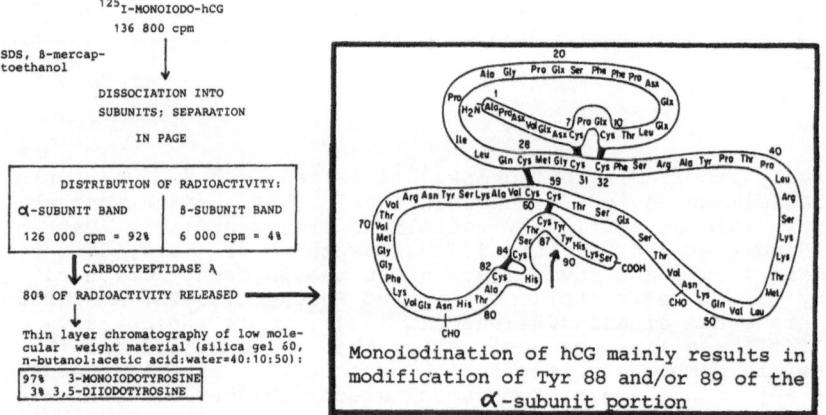

Monoiodination of hCG mainly results in modification of Tyr 88 and/or 89 of the α-subunit portion

Fig. 11. Localization of iodinated residues in monoiodo-hCG and quantification of the ratio of monoiodo:diiodotyrosine. Figure in insert shows structure of hCG-α-subunit according to Mise and Bahl (198o), with permission.

iodo-hCG measured in radioligand receptor assay, however, appears to be reduced by about 5o%, and is further diminished if additional iodine residues are introduced into the hCG molecule. At the moment it cannot be explained why monoiodo-hCG exhibits a higher biological activity in vivo (rat prostate assay) than in radioligand receptor test. One may speculate that deiodases in vivo are able to accept protein-bound iodine as substrate and to deliver it. As pointed out above, the C-terminal region of the α-subunit is a most critical domain because a structural modification in this region may result in more or less distinct conformational changes which are the cause for a diminution or a loss of biological activity. Thus, hCG is iodinated at a vulnerable point. This is due to the extraordinary reactivity of tyrosine residues 88, 89 at the C-terminus of the α-subunit portion. Ketelslegers and coauthors (1975) and Catt et al. (1976) also described that

Table 4. Biological activity of iodinated choriogonadotropin.

Biological activity in vivo (rat prostate assay) determined by
increase in weight of accessory reproductive organs of infantile
rats. Radioligand receptor assay applied for estimation of binding
activity in vitro using rat testes homogenate.

Protein	Rat prostate assay		Radioligand receptor assay	
	IU/mg	95% Confidence limits	IU/mg	95% Confidence limits
Native hCG	11 1oo	8 2oo - 14 9oo	1o ooo	9 1oo - 11 1oo
Monoiodo-hCG	9 2oo	6 6oo - 12 1oo	4 7oo	4 1oo - 5 3oo
Diiodo-hCG	n.d.[a]		3 ooo	2 3oo - 3 8oo
Pentaiodo-hCG	1 7oo	1 3oo - 2 3oo	43o	38o - 49o

[a]not determined

Table 5. Effect of iodination by lactoperoxidase method on binding
properties of choriogonadotropin (hCG) to Leydig cell receptors.

1.5 mg hCG dissolved in 25o µl o.2 M sodium phosphate buffer pH 7.2
iodinated in presence of 1.3 fold molar excess of NaI, solid phase
lactoperoxidase-glucose oxidase (Biorad, Munich) and 14 µmoles β-D-
glucose; total volume 79o µl; incubation time 3o Min, room tempera-
ture. Separation of reaction products by gel filtration on Sephadex G 25 column.

Protein	Iodine incorporated	Receptor binding activity[a]	95% Confidence limits	Precision
	mol	IU/mg		λ
Native hCG	-	12 3oo	11 1oo - 13 65o	o.o695
Control preparation[b]	-	11 79o	1o 27o - 13 6oo	o.o695
Monoiodo-hCG	1.o2	7 13o	6 37o - 8 o4o	o.o939

[a]Radioligand receptor assay, rat testes homogenate.
[b]Native hCG exposed to reagents without addition of sodium iodide.

the activity of ^{125}I-labelled hCG in radioligand receptor assay was
diminished. They attributed this to side reactions which result in
protein damage. We could not find, however, any hints of a heterogeneity of nonradioactively monoiodinated hCG. The potency of monoiodo-hCG
to bind to rat Leydig cell receptors is also diminished by more than
4o% when the modification is carried out applying the lactoperoxidase
method (Table 5) which allows a very mild oxidation. A control preparation of hCG which was exposed to reactants without addition of sodium iodide, however, is completely active, indicating that introduction of iodine itself into hCG molecule causes the lower receptor
binding ability.

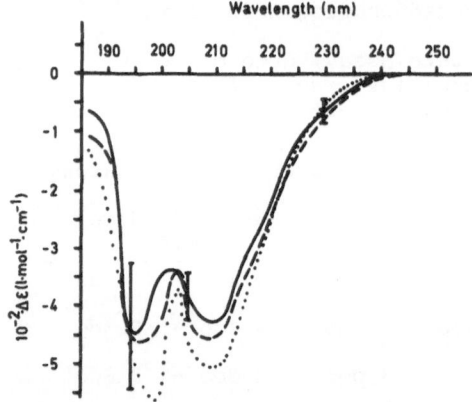

Fig. 12. Far ultraviolet circular dichroism of native hCG (——), monoiodo-hCG (— —), and pentaiodo-hCG (·······).
Protein concentration 1 mg/ml, o.1 M phosphate buffer pH 7, 20°C. Vertical bars extend to the oscillation range of CD signal.

The CD spectrum of monoiodinated hCG (Fig. 12) shows some minor differences in the far ultraviolet region especially in the absorption range of aperiodic structure which become more pronounced in the spectrum of pentaiodo-hCG. This result was to be expected from our investigations on CD of hCG with shortened C-terminus of the α-subunit portion (Merz 1979): We could find evidence for small conformational changes induced by modification of this region which are hardly visible in CD spectrum.
Monoiodo-hCG shows a significantly reduced potency to enhance ANS fluorescence whereas the iodine-free control preparation and native hCG display no difference. (Table 6). In presence of ANS, monoiodo-hCG aggregates uniformly without any differences from native hormone,

Table 6. Fluorescence of complexes of iodinated choriogonadotropin and 1-anilinonaphthalene-8-sulfonate (ANS).

Fluorescence at 489 nm, excitation wavelength 39o nm; ANS concentration 2o μM (Mg^{2+} salt); final concentration of protein 1-2 nM.

Protein	Mol iodine incorporated /mol hCG	ANS / hCG fluorescence ± S.D. (n=6) %
Native hCG	-	1oo.o
HCG control[a]	-	94.3 ± 2.o
Monoiodo-hCG	o.9	45.5 ± o.5
Pentaiodo-hCG	4.9	24.3 ± 1.3

[a] HCG, treated with chloramin T and sodium metadisulfite in absence of iodine.

indicating that diminished fluorescence of complexes of ANS and monoiodo-hCG are probably not caused by a loss of binding sites for the ligand. Therefore, small conformational changes are most likely induced by monoiodination of hCG.
Immunological properties do not seem to be affected by monoiodination of hCG when tested with antisera in complement fixation assay or in radioimmunoassay.

The following conclusions can be drawn from iodination experiments
of hCG:
1) Monoiodination of hCG results in modification of the tyrosine residues 88 and/or 89 of the C-terminal region of the α-subunit portion.
2) This causes small conformational changes and a diminution of ability to bind to rat Leydig cell receptors.
3) Thus, observations of hormone receptor interactions obtained with
[125]I-labelled hCG possibly do not reflect the physiological situation.
4) When ^{125}I-labelled hCG is used for studies of the degradation of
the hormone, the catabolic velocity merely of the C-terminus of the
α-subunit portion is followed up because the hormone is labelled at
a single point in a region which is readily accessible to proteolytic
enzymes (e.g. carboxypeptidases).

PEPTIDE REGIONS OF THE hCG-α-SUBUNIT "BURIED" OR LOCATED ON SURFACE

The enzymatic and chemical modifications discussed above as well as
a variety of other modifications of hCG or LH carried out in this laboratory and by others (recently reviewed by Pierce and Parsons 1981)
e.g. chemical modification of methionine residues (Cheng 1976a,b;
Merz 1977; Merz 1980), tyrosine residues (Brossmer et al. 1969;
Brossmer et al. 1971; Sairam et al. 1972; Cheng and Pierce 1972;
Hum et al.1974; Liu and Ward 1975; Hum et al. 1976; Brossmer and Merz
1976; Merz 1977; Merz 1980), histidine residues (Aggarwal and Papkoff
1979; Merz 1980), and disulfide bonds (Giudice and Pierce 1976;
Pierce et al. 1976) can be used for a rough classification of peptide
regions which probably are located at the surface of the isolated α-
subunit and those hidden in the inner part of the molecule (Fig. 13).
The superficially arranged residues or peptide regions are easily
accessible to chemical reagents, enzymatic attack, and also antibodies.
They provide contact areas for interactions with β-subunit and perhaps with parts of receptor molecules of target cells. Information
about the precise orientation of each amino acid residue, however,
cannot be deduced from this simple model. This is left to X-ray structure analysis. As pointed out above, the region comprising the residues 30-50 does not seem to be accessible to trypsin and chymotrypsin
in native hCG in contrast to the isolated α-subunit. Therefore, in
accordance with Pierce and Parsons (1981) it is concluded that the
binding area for the β-subunit is located in this region. The C-terminal region of the α-subunit is arranged on the surface and thus
accessible to chemical reagents and enzymes in the isolated subunit
as well as in the hCG molecule. This region is essential for the biological properties of hCG, LH and TSH (Cheng et al. 1973; Merz 1979;
Parsons and Pierce 1979; Merz and Dörner 1979; Merz and Dörner 1983).
Some antigenic determinants of the isolated subunit are located in
the N-terminal region (Parlow and Shome 1975). This classification of
peptide regions must also be discussed in regard to the distribution
of polar and apolar amino acid residues along the sequence of the α-
subunit (Fig. 14). The polarity profile of the hCG-α-subunit shows
two contrary peptide regions: a very hydrophobic region near the N-
terminus and a hydrophilic domain. This distribution was highly conserved during evolution which is evident from a comparison of polarity profiles of bovine TSH-α- and hCG-α-subunits indicating that the
antagonism of extended hydrophilic and hydrophobic regions is an essential element of α-subunit structure. The carbohydrate chains
are situated in the hydrophilic part. Tyrosines 88, 89 and 65 are located in hydrophilic domains and therefore can be chemically modified,
whereas Tyr 37 seems to be buried though it is in the neighbourhood
of peptide bonds which are readily hydrolyzed by trypsin.

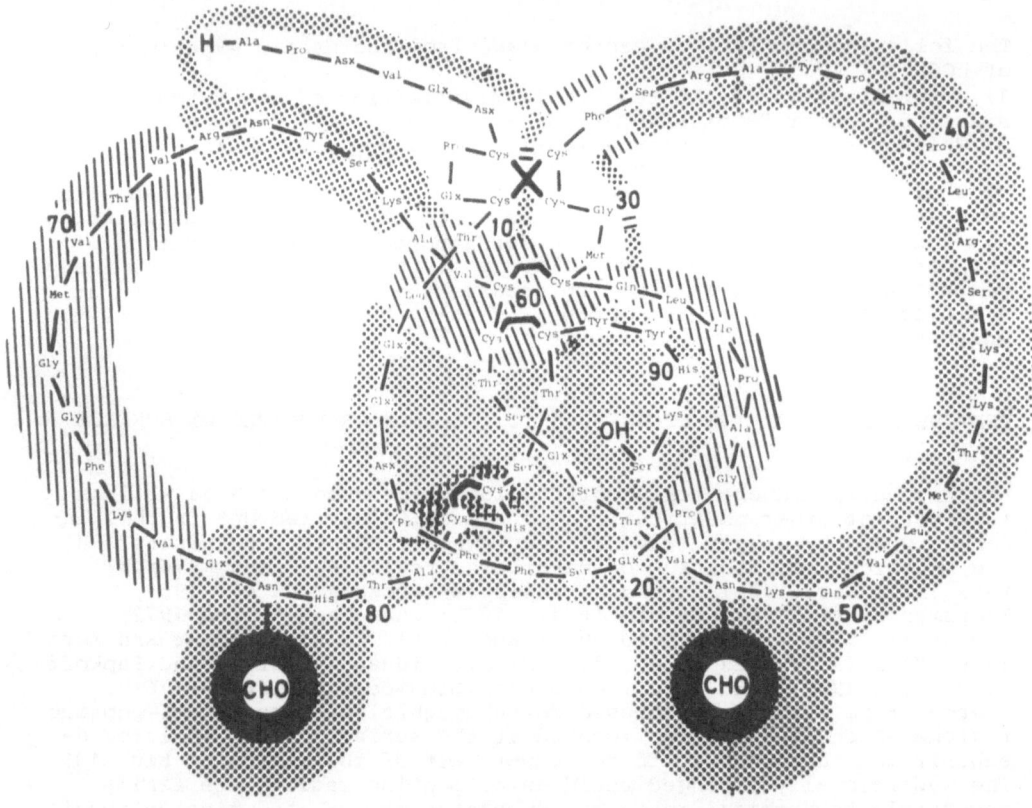

Fig. 13. Model of the hCG-α-subunit which shows peptide regions probably situated at the surface of the isolated subunit (dotted areas)
and inside the molecule (hatched areas), respectively. The N-terminal
region is most probably arranged at the surface, the coordination of
the region around disulfide bridges between the cysteine residues
7-31 and 1o-32 is uncertain. Arrangement of disulfide bonds according to Mise and Bahl (198o).

BIOSYNTHESIS OF hCG

Recently we have started to investigate the biosynthesis of hCG in
placental tissue culture in presence of radioactive amino acids or
carbohydrates (Hilf et al. 1982). The structure of radioactive hCG obtained by biosynthesis in tissue culture is not altered by chemical
modification. We intend to use this hormone to study its molecular
properties and the internalization and degradation in target cells.
Biosynthesis is measured by means of radioactivity incorporated in
immunoprecipitated hCG or subunits. Secretion of hCG or isolated subunits is determined from the content of these compounds in culture
medium with hCG - or subunit - specific radioimmunoassays. In Fig. 15
the time course of biosynthesis and secretion of hCG in 4 different
placental cultures and the influence of cAMP is depicted. It is known
from literature that dibutyryl-cAMP enhances hCG biosynthesis (Hussa
1977; Hussa et al. 1978; Chou et al. 1978; Huot et al. 1979; Haning
et al. 1982; Hilf et al. 1982), but we were greatly astonished to see

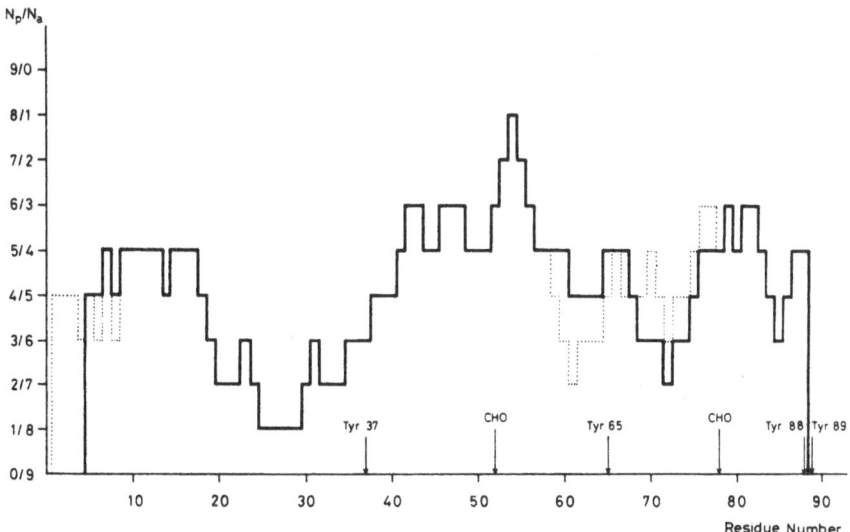

Fig. 14. Plots of the ratio between the number of polar (N_p) and apolar (N_a) residues in nonapeptide segments of the α-subunits of hCG (solid line) and bovine TSH (dotted line). Each ratio was plotted at the central residue of the respective nonapeptide. CHO = carbohydrate residue of hCG-α-subunit. Sequence data taken from Bellisario et al (1973). Classification of amino acids according to Edmundson et al. (1973).

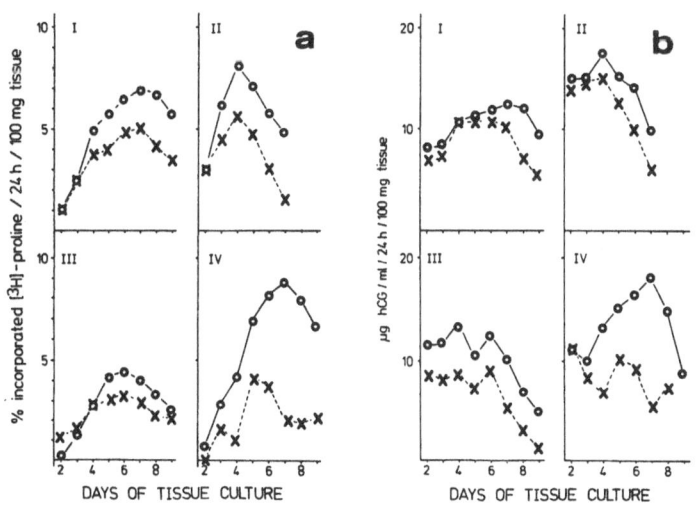

Fig. 15. Influence of cAMP (1 mM) (O) and dibutyryl-cAMP (1 mM) (X) in presence of IBMX (0.1 mM) on hCG biosynthesis and secretion in culture of placental tissue (7–9 weeks gestational age) of 4 different donors. a: Specific incorporation of L- $[5-^3H]$ -proline into hCG. Radioactivity measured in immunoprecipitated hCG. b: Secreted hCG in culture medium determined by radioimmunoassay.

that cAMP is even superior to dibutyryl-cAMP. Closer inspection showed that cAMP induces an optimum secretion of hCG twice as high as found in cultures without the addition of cAMP and IBMX (Fig. 16). The amount of isolated subunits is low in our tissue cultures (< 10% w/w of secreted amount of hCG) and no excessive secretion of a single subunit is observed. It is known from several investigations that the genetic information for biosynthesis of hCG α- and β-subunits is encoded in distinct genes (Daniels-McQueen et al. 1978; Godine et al. 1982; Boorstein et al. 1982). The process of subunit assembly is un- known. A preliminary result gives rise to some speculations on the in- fluence of cAMP and IBMX on biosynthesis and secretion of the α-sub- unit: In Figure 16a it is shown that addition of IBMX to culture me- dium increases the amount of secreted hCG. In the presence of IBMX + cAMP highest concentrations of secreted hCG are obtained. When the ratio of secreted hCG versus secreted α-subunit is plotted, marked effects were observed (Fig. 16b): In the presence of cAMP the total secretion of hCG rises at the expense of α-subunit secretion. In this case the ratio of hCG versus α-subunit is lower than in cultures without additives. The effects on the hCG/β-subunit ratio are less pronounced. Therefore it is tempting to speculate that the activity of the α-subunit gene is regulated in a more flexible way, and might be influenced by cAMP. Thus the α-subunit might regulate hCG bio-

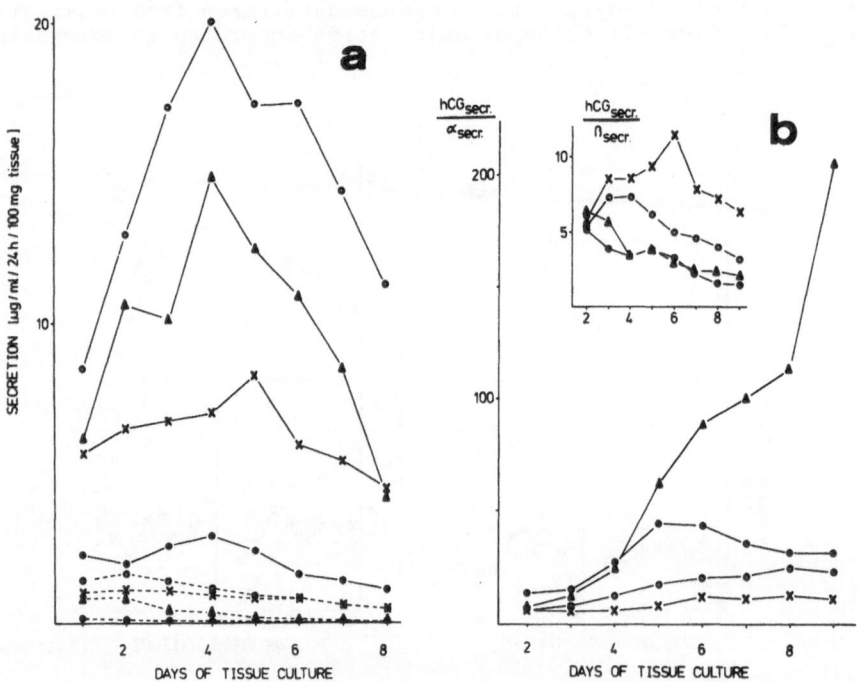

Fig. 16. Influence of IBMX (0.1 mM) (▲) and IBMX in combination with cAMP (1 mM) (O) or dibutyryl-cAMP (1 mM) (X) on hCG (solid line) or hCG-α-subunit (dotted line) content of medium of placental tissue cul- ture (a) and ratios of hCG and isolated hCG-subunits (b). Results of tissue culture in absence of IBMX, dibutyryl-cAMP, and cAMP (●).

synthesis via the process of subunit assembly. The tremendous effect
of IBMX on hCG/α ratio shown here could not be reproduced in all cases
and needs further investigations.
The initial questions concerning the function of the α-subunit may be
answered in the following way:
1) The regulating function of the α-subunit in biosynthesis of hCG is
not yet understood. Biosynthesis of β-subunit is reported to be rate-
limiting for hCG biosynthesis (Daniels-McQueen et al. 1978). In some
cases, however, e.g. in DoT and CaSki cell lines the α-subunit seems
to control the rate of hCG biosynthesis (Cole et al. 1981). Our findings described above seem to indicate that this also might occur in
placental tissue culture.
2) It was shown that the α-subunit interacts with the β-subunit in a
manner which causes structural organization of specific receptor binding sites.
3) There is no indication for receptor binding being directly mediated
by the α-subunit.
The thesis No. 4, the α-subunit might be directly involved in mediation of hormone activity, is open to speculations and a challenge for
further studies.

ACKNOWLEDGMENTS

The investigations were supported by the Deutsche Forschungsgemeinschaft, Bonn - Bad Godesberg. I am indebted to Anna Lorenzen for the
revision of the english manuscript, and to Hilde Anslinger for typing
the manuscript. The radioimmunological studies were performed in part
in cooperation with Dr. M. Dörner. The technical assistance of Mrs. U.
Langula is gratefully acknowledged.

REFERENCES

Aggarwal BB, Papkoff H (1979) Role of histidine residues in ovine
    lutropin: Effects on steroidogenic activity. Biochem Biophys Res
    Comm 89:169-174
Aloj SM, Edelhoch H, Ingham KC, Morgan FJ, Ganfield RE, Ross GT (1973a)
    The rates of dissociation and reassociation of the subunits of human
    chorionic gonadotropin. Arch Biochem Biophys 159:497-5o4
Aloj SM, Ingham KC, Edelhoch H (1973b) Interaction of 1,8-ANS with
    human luteinizing hormones: A probe for subunit interactions of
    hCG and hLH. Arch Biochem Biophys 155:478-479
Amr S, Wehman RE, Birken S, Canfield RE, Nisula BC (1983) Characteri-
    zation of a carboxyterminal peptide fragment of the human chorio-
    gonadotropin β-subunit excreted in the urine of a woman with
    choriocarcinoma. J Clin Invest 71:329-339
Amsterdam A, Nimrod A, Lamprecht SA, Burstein Y, Lindner HR (1979)
    Internalization and degradation of receptor-bound hCG in granulosa
    cell cultures. Am J Physiol 236:E129-E138
Amsterdam A, Naor Z, Knecht M, Dufau ML, Catt KJ (1981) Hormone action
    and receptor redistribution in endocrine target cells: Gonadotropins
    and gonadotropin-releasing hormone. In: Middlebrook JL, Kohn LD
    (eds) Receptor mediated binding and internalization of toxins and
    hormones. Acad Press, New York San Francisco London, pp 283-31o

and the activation of steroidogenesis in Leydig tumor cells. In:
Middlebrook JL, Kohn LD (eds) Receptor-mediated binding and internalization of toxins and hormones. Acad Press, New York San Francisco London, pp 271-281

Bellisario R, Carlsen RB, Bahl OP (1973) Human chorionic gonadotropin.
Linear amino acid sequence of the α-subunit. J Biol Chem 248:
6796-68o9

Bewley TA, Sairam MR, Li CH (1974) The kinetics of dissociation and
reassociation of ovine pituitary interstitial cell stimulating
hormone. Arch Biochem Biophys 163:625-633

Birken S, Canfield RE (1977) Isolation and amino acid sequence of COOH-
terminal fragments from the β-subunit of human choriogonadotropin.
J Biol Chem 252:5386-5392

Birken S, Canfield RE (198o) Chemistry and immunochemistry of human
chorionic gonadotropin. In: Segal,SJ (ed) Chorionic gonadotropin.
Plenum Press, New York London, pp 65-86

Boorstein WR, Vamvakopoulos NC, Fiddes JC (1982) Human chorionic gonadotropin β-subunit is encoded by at least eight genes arranged in
tandem and inverted pairs. Nature 3oo:419-422

Brand L, Gohlke JR, Rao DS (1967) Evidence for binding of rose bengal
and anilinonaphthalenesulfonates at the active site regions of liver
alcohol dehydrogenase. Biochemistry 6:351o-3518

Brossmer R, Trude E, Leidenberger F (1969) Purification and chemical
modification of human chorionic gonadotropin. 6th FEBS-Meeting,
Madrid, Abstr 811, p 255

Brossmer R, Dörner M, Hilgenfeldt U, Leidenberger F, Trude E (1971)
Chemical modification of human chorionic gonadotropin and its biological and immunological characterization. FEBS Lett 15:36-39

Brossmer R, Merz WE (1976) Carbohydrates and the biological function of
gonadotropin hormones. In: James VHT (ed) Proc V Intern Congr
Endocrinol, Hamburg, vol I. Excerpta Medica, Amsterdam, pp 92-98

Canfield RE, Morgan FJ, Kammerman S, Bell JJ, Agosto GM (1971) Studies
on Human chorionic gonadotropin. Recent Prog Horm Res 27:121-164

Carlsen RB, Bahl OP, Swaminathan N (1973) Human chorionic gonadotropin.
Linear amino acid sequence of the β-subunit. J Biol Chem 248:681o-
6827

Catt KJ, Tsuruhara T, Dufau ML (1972) Gonadotropin binding sites of the
rat testis. Biochim Biophys Acta 279:194-2o1

Catt KJ, Dufau ML, Tsuruhara T (1973) Absence of intrinsic biological
activity in LH and hCG subunits. J Clin Endocrinol Metab 36:73-8o

Catt KJ, Ketelslegers J-M, Dufau ML (1976) Receptors for gonadotropic
hormone. In: Blecher M (ed) Methods in receptor research, vol I.
Marcel Dekker Inc, New York Basel, pp 175-25o

Catt KJ, Dufau ML (1978) Gonadotropin receptors and regulation of in-
terstitial cell function in the testis. In: Birnbaumer L, O'Malley
BW (eds) Receptor and hormone action, vol III. Acad Press, New York
San Francisco London, pp 291-339

Catt KJ, Harwood JP, Clayton RN, Davies TF, Chan V, Katikineni M,
Nozu K, Dufau ML (198o) Regulation of peptide hormone receptors and
gonadal steroidogenesis. Recent Prog Horm Res 36:557-622

Cheng KW, Pierce JG (1972) The reaction of tetranitromethane with
pituitary, luteinizing and thyroid-stimulating hormone. J Biol
Chem 247:7163-7172

Cheng KW, Glazer AN, Pierce JG (1973) The effects of modification of
the COOH-terminal regions of bovine thyrotropin and its subunits.
J Biol Chem 248:793o-7937

Cheng KW (1976a) Carboxymethylation of methionine residues in bovine
pituitary luteinizing hormone and its subunits. Effects on the binding activity with receptor sites and interactions between subunits.
Biochem J 159:71-77

Cheng KW (1976b) Carboxymethylation of methionine residues in bovine pituitary luteinizing hormone and its subunits. Localization of specifically modified methionine residues. Biochem J 159:79-87

Cheung HC, Morales MF (1969) Studies on myosin conformation by fluorescent techniques. Biochemistry 8:2177-2182

Chou JY, Wang S-S, Robinson JC (1978) Regulation of the synthesis of human chorionic gonadotropin by 5-bromo-2'deoxyuridine and dibutyryl cyclic AMP in trophoblastic and nontrophoblastic tumor cells. J Clin Endocrinol Metab 47:46-51

Cody V, Hazel J (1977) Molecular conformation of 8-anilino-1-naphthalenesulfonate hemihydrate. A fluorescence probe for thyroxine binding globulin. J Medicin Chem 2o:12-17

Cole LA, Hussa RO, Rao CV (1981) Discordant synthesis and secretion of human chorionic gonadotropin and subunits by cervical carcinoma cells. Cancer Res 41:1615-1619

Daniels-McQueen S, McWilliams D, Birken S, Canfield RE, Landefeld T, Boime I (1978) Identification of mRNAs encoding the α and β subunits of human choriogonadotropin. J Biol Chem 253:71o9-7114

Dufau ML, Horner KA, Hayashi K, Tsuruhara T, Conn PM, Catt KJ (1978) Actions of choleragen and gonadotropin in isolated Leydig cells. Functional compartimentalization of hormone-activated cyclic AMP response. J Biol Chem 253:3721-3729

Edmundson AB, Schiffer M, Ely KR, Wood MK (1973) Structural features of immunoglobulin light chains. In: Hahn FF, Puck TT, Springer CF, Szybalski W, Wallenfels K (eds) Prog Mol Subcell Biology. Springer, Berlin Heidelberg New York, pp 159-182

Franchimont P, Hendrick JC, Reuter A, Legros JJ (1971) The gonadotropins: Radioimmunoassay technique and physiologic evidence of specificity. In: Saxena BB, Beling CG, Gandy HM (eds) Gonadotropins. Wiley-Interscience, New York London Sydney Toronto, pp 361-376

Giudice LC, Pierce JG (1976) Studies on the disulfide bonds of glycoprotein hormones. Complete reduction and reoxidation of the disulfide bonds of the α subunit of bovine luteinizing hormone. J Biol Chem 251:6392-6399

Godine JE, Chin WW, Habener JF (1982) Detection of two precursors to each of the subunits of human chorionic gonadotropin translated from placental mRNA in the wheat germ cell-free system. Biochem Biophys Res Comm 1o4:463-473

Haning jr RV, Choi L, Kiggens AJ, Kuzma DL, Summerville JW (1982) Effects of dibutyryl adenosine 3',5'-monophosphate, luteinizing hormone-releasing hormone, and aromatase inhibitor on simultaneous outputs of progesterone, 17 β-estradiol, and human chorionic gonadotropin by term placental explants. J Clin Endocrinol Metab 55:213-218

Hilf G, Merz WE, Schmidt W (1982) Biosynthesis and secretion of choriogonadotropin in placental tissue culture. Hoppe-Seyler's Z Physiol Chem 363:1o3o

Hum VG, Knipfel JE, Mori KF (1974) Human chorionic gonadotropin, reaction with tetranitromethane. Biochemistry 13:2359-2364

Hum VG, Botting H, Mori KF (1976) Human chorionic gonadotropin: Acetylation of tyrosyl with N-acetimidazole. Endocr Res Comm 3:145-156

Huot RI, Foidart J-M, Stromberg K (1979) Effects of culture conditions on the synthesis of human chorionic gonadotropin by placental organ cultures. In Vitro 15:497-5o2

Hussa RO (1977) Immunologic and physical characterization of human chorionic gonadotropin and its subunits in cultures of human malignant trophoblast. J Clin Endocrinol Metab 44:1154-1162

Hussa RO, Pattillo RA, Ruckert ACF, Scheuermann KW (1978) Effects of butyrate and dibutyryl cyclic AMP on hCG-secreting trophoblastic and non-trophoblastic cells. J Clin Endocrinol Metab 46:69-76

Ingham KC, Aloj SM, Edelhoch H (1974) Rates of dissociation and recombination of bovine thyrotropin. Arch Biochem Biophys 163:589-599

Ingham KC, Saroff HA, Edelhoch H (1975) Ligand-induced self-associa-
tion of human chorionic gonadotropin. Positive cooperativity in the
binding of 8-anilino-1-naphthalenesulfonate. Biochemistry 14:4751-
4758
Ingham KC, Weintraub BD, Edelhoch H (1976) Kinetics of recombination
of the subunits of human chorionic gonadotropin. Biochemistry 15:
172o-1726
Ingham KC, Bolotin C (1978) Intrinsic and extrinsic fluorescence probes of subunit interactions in ovine lutropin. Arch Biochem Biophys
191:134-145
Jonas A, Weber G (1971) Presence of arginin residues at the strong,
hydrophobic anion binding sites of bovine serum albumin. Biochemistry 1o:1335-1339
Kennedy JF, Chaplin MF (1976) The structures of the carbohydrate
moieties of the α subunit of human chorionic gonadotropin. Biochem
J 155:3o3-315
Kessler MJ, Reddy MS, Shah RH, Bahl OP (1979a) Structures of N-glycosidic carbohydrate units of human chorionic gonadotropin. J Biol
Chem 254:79o1-79o8
Kessler MJ, Mise T, Ghai RD, Bahl OP (1979b) Structure and location of
the O-glycosidic carbohydrate units of human chorionic gonadotropin.
J Biol Chem 254:79o9-7914
Ketelslegers J-M, Knott GD, Catt KJ (1975) Kinetics of gonadotropin
binding by receptors of the rat testis. Analysis by a nonlinear
curve-fitting method. Biochemistry 14:3o75-3o83
Keutmann HT, Williams (1977) Human chorionic gonadotropin. Amino acid
sequence of the hormone-specific COOH-terminal region. J Biol Chem
252:5393-5397
Leidenberger F, Reichert jr LE (1972a) Evaluation of a rat testis homogenate radioligand receptor assay for human pituitary LH. Endocrinology 91:9o1-9o9
Leidenberger F, Reichert jr LE (1972b) Studies on the uptake of human
chorionic gonadotropin and its subunits by rat testicular homoge-
nates and interstitial tissue. Endocrinology 91:135-143
Liu W-K, Ward DN (1976) Effect of selective nitration of ovine lutropin on the subunit association and biological activity of the hormone. J Biol Chem 251:316-319
Matsuura S, Ohashi M, Chen H-C, Hodgen GD (1979) A human chorionic
gonadotropin-specific antiserum against synthetic peptide analogs
to the carboxyl-terminal peptide of its β-subunit. Endocrinology
1o4:396-4o1
Merz WE, Hilgenfeldt U, Brockerhoff P, Brossmer R (1973) The time
course of recombination of human chorionic gonadotropin subunits
studied with immunological methods, circular-dichroic measurements
and bioassay. Eur J Biochem 35:297-3o6
Merz WE, Hilgenfeldt U, Brossmer R, Rehberger G (1974a) Amino acid
and carbohydrate composition of human chorionic gonadotropin frac-
tions obtained by isoelectric focusing. Hoppe-Seyler's Z Physiol
Chem 355:1o46-1o5o
Merz WE, Hilgenfeldt U, Dörner M, Brossmer R (1974b) Biological, immunological and physical investigations on human chorionic gonadotropin. Hoppe-Seyler's Z Physiol Chem 355:1o35-1o45
Merz WE (1977) Studies of structure function relationship of human
choriogonadotropin. Biological, immunological and physico-chemical
investigations. Thesis for habilitation, Fakultät für Naturwissen-
schaftliche Medizin, University of Heidelberg, pp 1-395
Merz WE (1979) Studies of the specific role of the subunits of choriogonadotropin for biological, immunological and physical properties
of the hormone. Digestion of the α-subunit with carboxypeptidase A.
Eur J Biochem 1o1:541-553
Merz WE, Dörner M (1979) Studies of the specific role of the subunits
of choriogonadotropin for biological, immunological and physical

properties of the hormone. Digestion of choriogonadotropin and its
isolated subunits with serine carboxypeptidase. Hoppe-Seyler's Z
Physiol Chem 36o:1783-1797

Merz WE (198o) Biological and physical properties of choriogonadotropin
(CG) containing a chemically modified α subunit. 13th FEBS Meeting
Jerusalem, Abstr C1o-P14

Merz WE, Sessler M (1981) Adenylcyclase-stimulating activity of enzymatically modified choriogonadotropin using rat Leydig cells purified by Percoll density gradient centrifugation. Acta endocr (Kbh)
96, suppl 24o:83-84

Merz WE, Dörner M (1983) Iodinated choriogonadotropin (hCG): Biological, physical and immunological investigations. Acta endocr 1o2,
suppl 253:51-52

Midgley jr AR, Pierce jr GB (1962) Immunohistochemical localization of
human chorionic gonadotropin. J exp Med 115:289-294

Mise T, Bahl OP (198o) Assignment of disulfide bonds in the α subunit
of human chorionic gonadotropin. J Biol Chem 255:8516-8522

Morgan FJ, Canfield RE, Vaitukaitis JL, Ross GT (1974) Properties of
the subunits of human chorionic gonadotropin. Endocrinology 94:
16o1-16o6

Morgan FJ, Birken S, Canfield RE (1975) The amino acid sequence of
human chorionic gonadotropin. The α and β subunit. J Biol Chem 25o:
5247-5258

Moss J, Vaughan M (1979) Activation of adenylate cyclase by choleragen.
Ann Rev Biochem 48:581-6oo

Müller WE (1976) The use of 8-anilino-1-naphthalene sulfonic acid as a
reporter group molecule for circular dichroism and fluorescence measurements. The effect of stearic acid and sodium dodecylsulfate on
the conformation of bovine and human serum albumin. Hoppe-Seyler's
Z Physiol Chem 357:1487-1494

Papkoff H, Li CH (197o) Studies on the chemistry of interstitial cell-
stimulating hormone. In: Butt WR, Crooke AC, Ryle M (eds) Gonadotropins and ovarian development. Livingstone, Edinburgh London, pp
138-148

Parlow AF, Shorne B (1975) A highly immunoreactive peptide fragment of
human luteinizing hormone alpha subunit, discerned with a new,
"sequence-specific" radioimmunoassay. J Clin Endocrinol Metab 41:
195-198

Parsons TF, Pierce JG (1979) Biologically active cross-linked glycoprotein hormones and the effect of modification of the COOH-terminal
region of their α subunits. J Biol Chem 254:6o1o-6o15

Pierce JG, Bahl OP, Cornell JS, Swaminathan N (1971) Biologically active hormones prepared by recombination of the α chain of human
chorionic gonadotropin and the hormone specific chain of bovine
thyrotropin or of bovine luteinizing hormone. J Biol Chem 246:
2321-2324

Pierce JG, Giudice LC, Reeve JR (1976) Studies on the disulfide bonds
of glycoprotein hormones. J Biol Chem 251:6388-6391

Pierce JG, Parsons TF (198o) Glycoprotein hormones: Similar molecules
with different functions. In: Sigman DS, Brazier MAB (eds) The evolution of protein structure and function. Acad Press, New York, pp
99-117

Pierce JG, Parsons TF (1981) Glycoprotein hormones: Structure and
function. Ann Rev Biochem 5o:465-495

Ramakrishnan S, Talwar (198o) Immuno-biological studies with beta-sub-
unit of human chorionic gonadotropin and its subfragments. In:
Segal SJ (ed) Chorionic gonadotropin. Plenum Press, New York London,
pp 213-23o

Rommerts FFG, Brinkman AO (1981) Modulation of steroidogenic activities
in testis Leydig cells. Mol Cell Endocrinol 21:15-28

Sairam MR, Papkoff H, Li CH (1972) Reaction of ovine interstitial cell stimulating hormone with tetranitromethane. Biochim Biophys Acta 278:421-432

Sairam MR, Chung D, Bewley TA, Li CH (1974) On the chemistry of pituitary interstitial cell stimulating hormone. In: Moudgal NR (ed) Gonadotropins and gonadal function. Acad Press, New York San Francisco London, pp 1-15

Saxena BB, Hasan SH, Haour F, Schmidt-Gollwitzer M (1974) Radioreceptor assay of human chorionic gonadotropin: Detection of early pregnancy. Science 184:793-795

Saxena BB (1976) Gonadotropin receptors. In: Blecher M (ed) Methods in receptor research, vol I. Marcel Dekker Inc, New York Basel, pp 251-299

Strickland TW, Puett D (1982) The kinetics and equilibrium parameters of subunit association and gonadotropin dissociation. J Biol Chem 257:2954-2960

Swaminathan N, Bahl OP (1970) Dissociation and recombination of the subunits of human chorionic gonadotropin. Biochem Biophys Res Comm 40:422-427

Talwar GP, Sharma NC, Dubey SK, Salahuddin M, Das C, Ramakrishnan S, Kumar S (1976) Isoimmunization against human chorionic gonadotropin with conjugates of processed β-subunit of the hormone and tetanus toxoid. Proc Natl Acad Sci USA 73:218-222

Vaitukaitis J, Robbins JB, Nieschlag E, Ross GT (1971) A method for producing specific antisera with small doses of immunogen. J Clin Endocr 33:988-991

Vaitukaitis JL, Ross GT, Braunstein GD, Rayford PL (1976) Gonadotropins and their subunits: Basic and clinical studies. Recent Prog Horm Res 32:289-331

Weber K, Osborn M (1969) The reliability of molecular weight determinations by dodecyl sulfate-polyacrylamide gel electrophoresis. J Biol Chem 244:4406-4412

Wildner GF (1976) The use of 1-anilino-8-naphthalene sulfonate as fluorescence probe for conformational studies on ribulose-1,5-bisphosphate carboxylase. Z Naturforsch 31c:267-271

Yoshinaga T (1976) Phosphoenolpyruvate carboxylase of Escherichia coli. Studies on multiple conformational states elicited by allosteric effectors with a fluorescent probe, 1-anilino-naphthalene-8-sulfonate. Biochim Biophys Acta 452:566-579

Phospholipid Turnover as a Mode of Gonadotropin Releasing Hormone Action in the Ovary

Z. Naor[1], N. Dekel[1], J. Molcho[2], Y. Eli[1], M. Zilberstein[2], and H. Zakut[2]

[1] Department of Hormone Research, The Weizmann Institute of Science, Rehovot 76100, Israel
[2] Sackler Faculty of Medicine, Tel Aviv University, The Edith Wolfson Hospital, Holon, Israel

INTRODUCTION

The extra-pituitary effects of GnRH and its analogs are well recognized by now (for review see Hsueh 1981; Knecht 1983). The anti-fertility effects exerted by GnRH analogs might be explained by desensitization of pituitary responsiveness to continuous challenge of the
hormone; by down-regulation of gonadal LH receptors and/or by direct
gonadal effects. In the female rat the anti-fertility effects exerted by GnRH agonistic analogs include: implantation delay and pregnancy termination; decrease in ovarian steroidogenesis and gonadotropin receptor content; inhibition of follicular maturation and
ovulation; decrease in uterine and oviductal growth; delay in puberty; delay of parturition and inhibition of ovarian steroid dependent
tumorigenesis (for review see Hsueh 1981). The inhibitory effects of
GnRH might be explained by recent findings that GnRH reverse the inhibitory effect of FSH on phosphodiesterase activity and progressive-
ly inhibit adenylate cyclase activity (Knecht 1981). Moreover, GnRH
inhibition of FSH-induced progesterone formation might result from
inhibition of the side-chain cleavage enzyme and the increase in 20-α
hydroxysteroid dehydrogenase activity (Jones, 1982).

Recently it was reported that GnRH exerts also stimulatory effects on
the ovary. The stimulatory effects include stimulation of prostaglandins (PG's) and progesterone production, resumption of meiosis of
follicle enclosed rat oocyte in vitro and induction of ovulation in
hypophysectomized (hypox) rats (Hillensjo 1980; Corbin 1981; Ekholm
1981; Dekel 1983). In this review we will focus on the stimulatory
effects of GnRH on gonadal functions. Specific gonadal high-affinity
binding sites were demonstrated for GnRH (Clayton 1979) indicating
that the effects described are receptor-mediated. Since GnRH exerted
both stimulatory and inhibitory effects it was thought that acute
treatment results in stimulation while chronic treatment will produce
inhibition of gonadal function (for review see Hsueh 1981). To check
this hypothesis we have used the 'super-ovulation' rat model.

Dissociation Between the Stimulatory and Inhibitory Effects of GnRH.

A single injection of [D-Ala^6]-des-Gly^{10}-GnRH N ethylamide (GnRHa,
2 μg/rat) was sufficient to obtain a 75% inhibition of hCG-induced
ovulation in PMSG-primed intact or hypox immature (26 days old) rats
(Naor 1983a). Inhibition of ovarian development in terms of growth
and ovulation by chronic administration of the analog (2 μg/rat twice
daily for 3 days) was achieved only when GnRHa was administered con-
comitantly with PMSG treatment (Fig. 1). When initiation of the
treatment with GnRHa was delayed after PMSG injection, stimulation
rather than inhibition occurred and the peptide induced ovulation

even in the absence of hCG treatment (Fig. 2). Under both regimes of
GnRHa administration the inhibitory (Fig. 1) or the stimulatory (Fig.
2), the oocytes of the treated rats were induced to resume meiosis
(Naor 1983a).

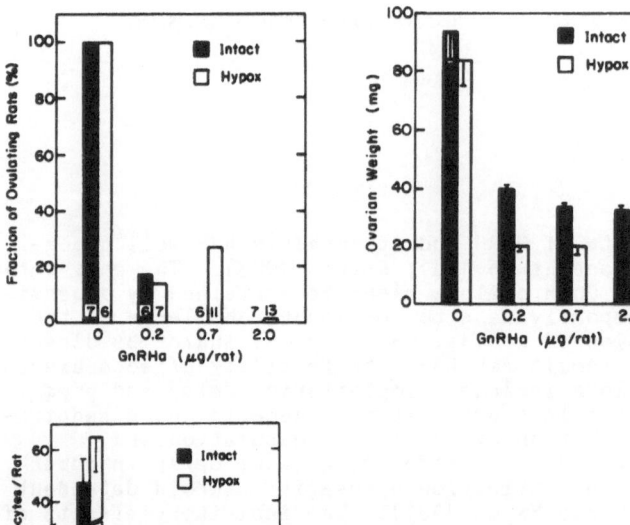

Fig. 1. Effect of GnRH agonist analog (injections twice daily) on
ovulation rate, number of ovulated oocytes and ovarian weight gain in
PMSG-primed (15 IU) hCG treated (5 and 10 IU in intact and hypox respectively) immature rats.

We therefore concluded that the follicular stage of development rather than the dose or duration of GnRHa administration determines
whether GnRHa inhibits or stimulates the ovary, while the competence
of the oocytes to respond to GnRH stimulus and resume meiosis is independent of hormonal priming (Naor 1983a).

A dissociation between the stimulatory and inhibitory effects of GnRH
at the ovarian level could be demonstrated in the intact rat as well
as in the hypophysectomized rat. However, the intact rat appeared to
be more sensitive, since a lower dose of GnRHa per rat was required
to obtain both its inhibitory and stimulatory actions. It is possible that elevation of endogenous LH, triggered by GnRHa in the intact
rats, contributes to the GnRHa stimulatory effect on the ovary and
also amplifies its inhibitory action, perhaps by causing down-regulation of gonadal LH receptors. In the male, the inhibitory effect of
GnRHa on testicular functions results primarily from increased endogenous LH levels (Seguin 1982).

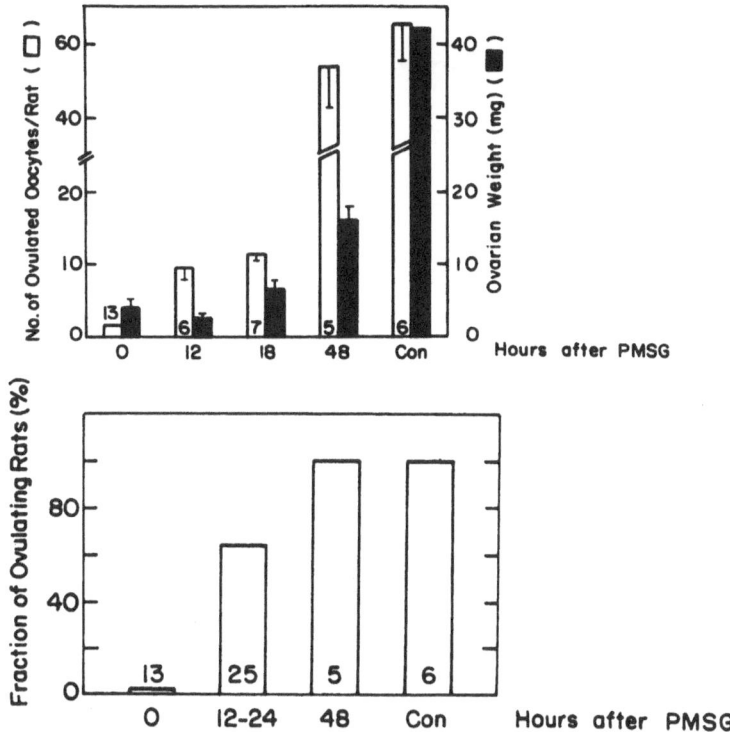

Fig. 2. Effect of delay in GnRHa administration on the fraction of
ovulating rats, the number of ovulated oocytes/rat and ovarian weight
gain in PMSG-primed hypox rats.

The molecular mechanisms underlying the extra-pituitary effects of
GnRH are not well understood. We therefore employed cultured granulosa cells to explore the direct effects of GnRH. Unlike LH, GnRH
does not stimulate cyclic AMP (cAMP) formation during a 4 h incubation period (Fig. 3). Since we have recently suggested that phospholipid turnover might be involved in GnRH induced gonadotropin release
(Naor 1981, 1983b), we decided to follow the possible involvement of
phospholipid turnover and PG's production in the ovarian actions of
GnRH and its analogs.

Phosphatidylinositol Turnover

Several ligand-receptor interactions results in increased phosphatidylinositol (PI) turnover (Fig. 4; and for review see Michell 1975).
The effect is specific to PI and phosphatidic acid (PA). It is remarkable in that the two phospholipids constitute only a small fraction of cellular phospholipids. In most cases the stimuli evoke an
increase in turnover rather than an increase in net synthesis of PI
and PA. The effect was first observed by the Hokin's (1953) and later regarded as a more general mechanism for ligand-receptor interaction (Michell 1975), in particular those involved in calcium mobilization and cyclic GMP production (e.g. adrenalin and acetylcholine).
It is interesting to note that in most systems where enhanced PI
turnover was reported, the effect could be observed in the absence of
calcium, indicating that the calcium-required step is at a postrecep-
tor locus after the PI effect.

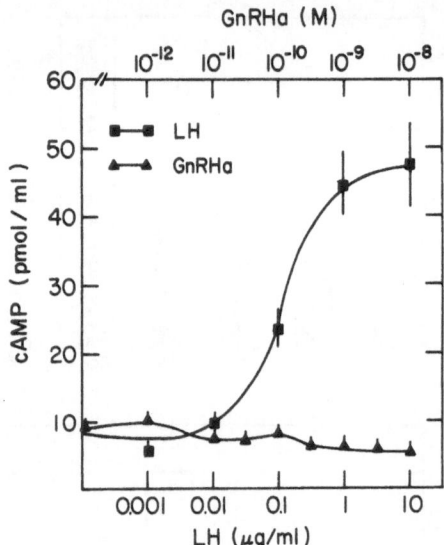

GnRHa (M)

Fig. 3. Effect of GnRHa and LH on cyclic AMP (cAMP) production (4 h) in cultured granulosa cells from preovulatory follicles.

Detection of enhanced labeling of PI and PA using ^{32}P-orthophosphate as a probe, ranges from 2 s in platelets, to 2-5 min in other target cells, and therefore can be regarded as one of the earliest steps in hormone action. Ligand-induced PI turnover might result in multiple phosphorylation of PI. The newly formed di- and triphosphoinositides were implicated in nervous conduction, in nicotinic cholinergic receptor activation (Michell 1975), and in mediating ACTH action on adrenal steroidogenesis (Farese 1980). Alteration of membrane phospholipid constituents might also result in changes in membrane fluidity, lateral mobility, coupling of hormone-receptor complex to the adenylate cyclase system, clustering and internalization of hormone-receptor complexes, desensitization and down-regulation (Cuatrecasas 1975; Rimon 1978; Strulovici 1981).

Another effect of phospholipid turnover and in particular the 'PI response' is the opening of calcium channels following receptor activation (Fain 1982). In most cases ligand-induced PI turnover is calcium-independent, and the enzyme that catalyses the formation of PI, CDP-diglyceride inositol transferase is inhibited by elevated Ca^{2+} in some tissues. Therefore, elevation of cytosolic Ca^{+} is secondary to PI breakdown in the plasma membrane, and PA was recently implicated as an endogenous calcium ionophore (Tyson 1976; Putney 1980; Salmon 1980).

Phosphaditylinositol turnover is also involved in prostaglandin formation. The diglyceride formed can be acted upon by a diglyceride lipase to liberate arachidonic acid (AA) that serves as the substrate for PG synthesis. In platelets the formation of PA precedes the release of AA from cellular phospholipids. Initially thrombin activates a PI-specific phospholipase C which converts PI to diacylglycerol. If the diglyceride escapes the lipase, it would be phosphorylated to PA. The phosphatidate thus formed serves as a calcium ionophore and activates a PA-specific phospholipase A_2 that liberate AA from PA. The phosphatidate and its residue lysophosphatidate induce further calcium gating and activate phospholipase A_2 that acts on other phospholipids to release more AA (Lapetina 1981, see Fig. 4). Thus, although PI is not a major phospholipid constituent, it is the main source of the AA needed for PG synthesis in platelets (Fain 1982).

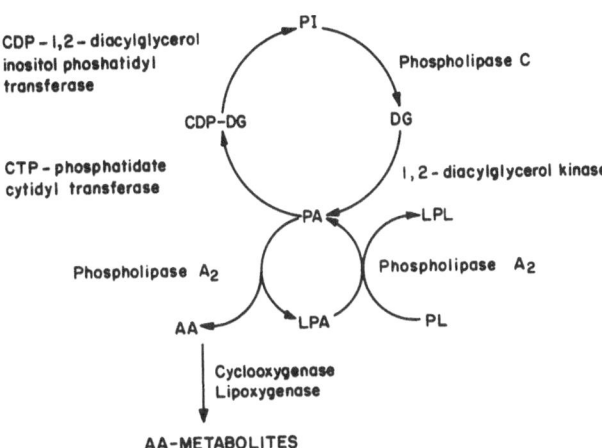

Fig. 4. Phosphatidylinositol (PI) cycle. Receptor activation results in breakdown of PI to 1,2-diacylglycerol (DG) by a PI-specific phospholipase C. Phosphorylation by ATP and activation by diacylglycerol kinase forms phosphatidic acid (PA). Conjugation with CTP by phosphatidic acid; CTP cytidyltransferase forms CDP-diacylglycerol (CDP-DG). The final reaction is an exchange of the activated CDP with free inositol by CDP-diacylglycerol inositol phosphatidyltransferase. The PA formed can be acted upon by a PA-specific phospholipase A_2 producing lysophosphatidic acid (LPA). Further calcium gating by LPA will stimulate phospholipase A_2 acting on other phospholipids (PL) to release more arachidonic acid (AA).

The diglyceride formed during PI-turnover can also activate a recently described cAMP-independent, calcium-dependent protein kinase C (Kishimoto 1980). This kinase initiates calcium-activated phosphorylation of key proteins and enzymes. Such a mechanism will link a receptor mediated event at the plasma membrane level, and biochemical reactions within the cell machinery that are dependent on phosphorylation-dephosphorylation.

It is interesting to note that PI turnover and calcium mobilization may be considered a major alternative pathway for peptide hormones which do not act via cyclic nucleotide production. For example, the hormones which activate hepatocyte glycogen phosphorylase can be divided to cAMP-dependent and cAMP-independent activators. Among the first group are glucagon and β-catecholamines and among the second group vasopressin, angiotensin and α-catecholamines. Those which do not increase cAMP levels are thought to activate PI turnover and elevate cytosolic calcium (Fain 1982).

Phospholipid Turnover and GnRH Action on the Ovary

Cultured ovarian granulosa cells from preantral or preovulatory follicles were prelabeled with [^{32}P]Pi to label endogenous phospholipids. After hormonal stimulation cellular phospholipids were extracted, separated on two-dimensional TLC, identified by autoradiog-
raphy and the radioactivity determined. GnRH and its analogs increased markedly the ^{32}P incorporation into phosphatidylinositol (PI)
and phosphatidic acid (PA) (Fig. 5; Naor 1982). The stimulatory effect of GnRHa was blocked by the potent GnRH antagonist
[D-pGlu^1,pclPhe^2, D-Trp^{3,6}]GnRH (kindly supplied by Dr. D. Coy,
U.S.A.) indicating that the effect was specific and receptor-mediated. In terms of the time course GnRH stimulated phospholipid labeling (5-10 min) represents the earliest biochemical response to the
hormone and hence might be responsible for initiating a cascade of
responses culminating in oocyte maturation and induction of ovulation
(Naor 1972; Dekel 1983).

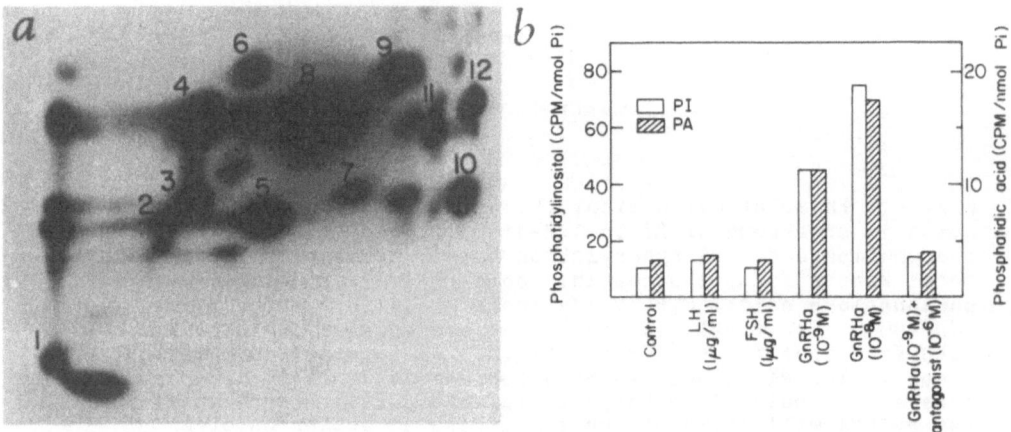

Fig. 5. a) Relative migration of ^{32}P-labeled phospholipids isolated
from cultured granulosa cells. Phospholipids were extracted and separated on two dimensional TLC. The numbers on the autoradiographs
denote the relative migration of the phospholipids: origin (1), uni-
dentified, possibly phosphatidylinositol plasmalogen (2), lysophos-
phatidylcholine (3), phosphatidylcholine plasmalogen (4), phosphatidylinositol (PI, 5), phosphatidylethanolamine plasmalogen (6)
phosphatidylserine (7), phosphatidylcholine (8), phosphatidylethanolamine (9), phosphatidic acid (PA, 10), phosphatidylglycerol (11),
cardiolipin (12).
b) Effect of GnRHa, LH, FSH and GnRH-antagonist on phospholipid labeling.

Increased PI turnover ('phospholipid effect') is believed to precede
the opening of calcium channels (Michell 1975) and phosphatidic acid
is believed to play a role of an endogenous calcium ionophore (Tyson
1976). We therefore propose that following its binding to specific
ovarian receptors (Clayton 1979) GnRH activates the phospholipid ef-

fect and elevates the levels of cytosolic calcium. Following the
opening of calcium channels phospholipase A_2 activity is increased
and arachidonic acid (AA) is liberated from cellular phosphoglycer-
ides (Fig. 4).

Since AA is not accumulated in the cell as a free fatty acid it is
rapidly esterified into cellular prostaglandins and leukotrienes.
Indeed in agreement with a recent report (Clark 1982), we found increased levels of prostaglandin E (PGE) after GnRHa stimulation of
cultured granulosa cells (Fig. 6). Both LH and GnRHa increase PGE
and progesterone production (Fig. 7) in granulosa cells with different time- and dose-response profiles (Zilberstein submitted). However, while cAMP mediates LH induced PGE and progesterone formation
(Zor 1977), we suggest that GnRH stimulated PGE production is derived
from increased PI turnover as is the case with angiotensin II action
in the kidney (Benabe 1982) and caerulein in the exocrine pancreas
(Marshall 1981).

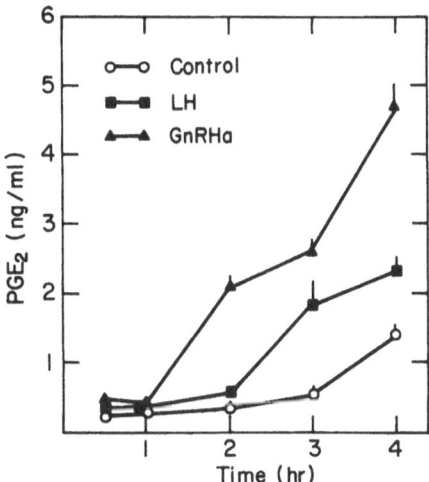

Fig. 6. Effect of GnRHa and LH on PGE formation in cultured granulosa cells. The cultured cells were incubated with oLH (1 μg/ml) and
GnRHa (10^{-7}M) for the time indicated and prostaglandin E_2 levels were
determined by RIA.

Recently, we have suggested that lipoxygenase products of AA might be
involved in GnRH action on pituitary gonadotropin release (Naor
1983b). In the ovary however, PG's seem to be the pathway of choice
for GnRH action. Therefore GnRH might be an example of a peptide
hormone capable of activating the different pathways of AA metabolism
(cyclooxygenase vs. lipoxygenase) in different target cells.

It is believed that LH-induced cAMP formation mediates also progesterone formation (Zor 1972). It is possible that GnRHa-stimulated PI
turnover is also involved in progesterone formation via the production of 1,2 diacylglycerol and activation of the recently discovered
calcium-dependent, phospholipid-activated protein kinase (Kishimoto
1980). Alternatively, it is possible that polyphosphoinositides derived from PI (DPI and TPI) are involved in GnRH-induced progesterone
formation in analogy to their role in adrenal steroidogenesis (Farese

1980). Nevertheless, we have excluded the possibility that PGE mediates LH- and GnRH-induced progesterone formation by demonstrating
that indomethacin had no inhibitory action on the peptide induced
progesterone formation (Zilberstein submitted).

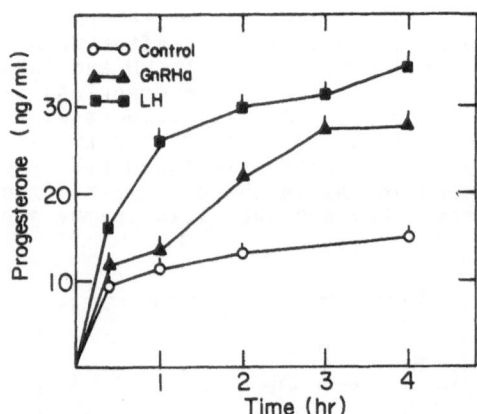

<u>Fig. 7.</u> Effect of GnRHa (10^{-7}M) and LH (1 μg/ml) on progesterone
formation. Granulosa cells were incubated with GnRHa and oLH for 4
h. Progesterone levels were measured in the medium by RIA.

Since GnRH mimics several actions of LH (PGE and progesterone formation; oocyte maturation and induction of ovulation) a mediatory role
for ovarian GnRH-like material in LH actions was considered. However, while a potent GnRH antagonist was capable of blocking stimulation of gonadal functions by GnRH, no inhibitory effect was noticed
on LH stimulation of oocyte maturation and induction of ovulation
(Fig. 8 and Dekel 1983).

Administration of indomethacin blocked the stimulatory effect of both
LH and GnRHa on induction of ovulation but had no inhibitory effect
on the peptide-induced oocyte maturation in vitro (Fig. 8). On the
other hand, we have recently shown that the stimulatory effect of LH
and GnRHa on resumption of meiosis in follicle-enclosed rat oocytes
in vitro was blocked by dibutyryl cAMP (DBC) and by MIX (Fig. 8 and
Dekel 1983). Prostaglandins of the E type (PGE) are involved in mediating LH effect on induction of ovulation but the exact mechanisms
involved in oocyte maturation are not yet understood. We suggest
here that the direct stimulatory effect of GnRH on oocyte maturation
and induction of ovulation are most likely mediated by a rapid PI
turnover followed by PGE and progesterone formation. In contrast, LH
stimulation of ovarian function is mediated by cAMP, PGE and progesterone production (Fig. 9). We therefore suggest that the initially
independent pathways of LH and GnRH converge at a step proximal to
PGE production and thereafter share similar pathways leading to oocyte maturation and independently to induction of ovulation (Fig. 9).

The stimulatory actions of GnRHa upon ovarian functions are most
likely calcium-dependent since PG synthesis is dependent on the presence of elevated calcium. Moreover, it was recently demonstrated
that the inhibitory effect of a GnRH agonist upon LH-induced cAMP

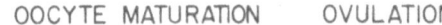

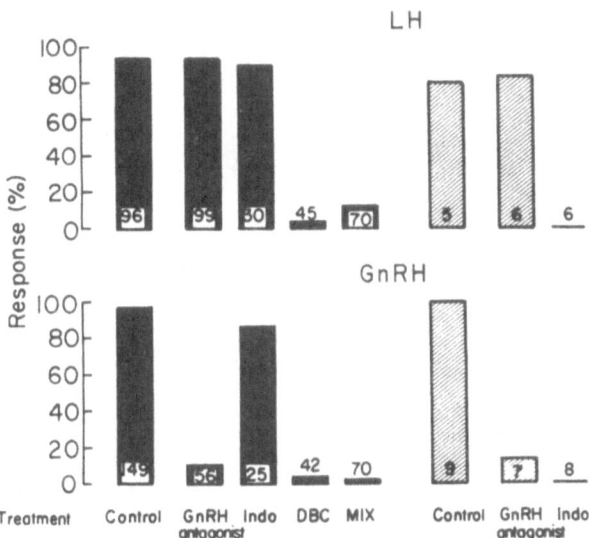

Fig. 8. Comparative studies on GnRH and LH stimulation of ovarian functions. To study oocyte maturation, follicles were isolated from the ovaries of immature rats 48 h after PMSG (15 IU/rat) priming and incubated in the presence of either oLH (0.1 μg/ml) or GnRHa (10^{-7}M) with or without either GnRH antagonist [D-pGlu^1, pclPhe^2, D-Trp^{3,6}]-GnRH, (10^{-5}M), dibutyryl cyclic AMP (DBC, 5 mM), MIX (0.2 mM) or indomethacin (Indo 10 μg/ml). The incidence of maturation was indicated by the breakdown of the germinal vesicles. Ovulation was studied in mature rats hypophysectomized and treated with PMSG (15 IU) on the morning of proestrus and 24 h later injected with hCG (4 IU/rat) or GnRHa (500 ng/rat) with or without a combined treatment with either GnRH antagonist (5 μg/rat) or indomethacin (2 mg/rat). The presence of ovulated oocytes was examined 20 h after hormonal treatment.

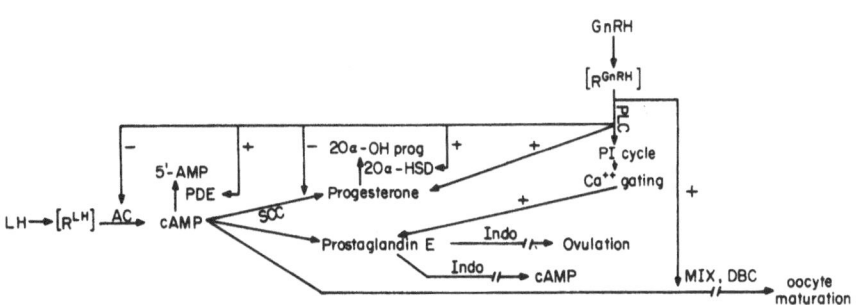

Fig. 9. Scheme of proposed mechanism of LH and GnRH action. R, represent the respective specific receptor for LH and GnRH; PI, phosphatidylinositol; indo, indomethacin; MIX, 3-isobutyl-1-methylxanthine; DBC, dibutyryl cAMP.

formation is completely dependent on extracellular calcium (Knecht 1983). Since GnRH-induced PI turnover precedes the previously de-scribed inhibitory and stimulatory actions of GnRH agonists upon the ovary (Naor 1982), it is possible that the PI turnover is responsible for calcium gating which mediates both inhibitory and stimulatory ac-tions of GnRH at the ovarian level.

The inhibitory effects apparently can be detected only after several hours of exposure to the hormone and are not observed during the ini-tial 4 h of incubation. Thus, binding of GnRH to its specific ovari-an receptors is followed by activated PI turnover and increased cal-cium fluxes (Fig. 9). The increased cytosolic calcium modulates adenylate cyclase and phosphodiesterase activities. Moreover the in-hibition of GnRH on FSH-induced progesterone formation might result from inhibition of the side chain cleavage enzyme and increase in 20α- hydroxysteroid dehydrogenase activity (Jones 1982). Collective-ly, the inhibitory effects are slow and can commence only after sev-eral hours of exposure to a GnRH challenge. On the other hand, we suggest that elevated calcium induced by GnRH via the phospholipid effect can stimulate phospholipase A_2 which leads to increased forma-tion of arachidonic acid and prostaglandin formation. The early res-ponses to GnRH agonists might therefore be involved in initiating a series of biochemical events that culminate in stimulatory and inhi-bitory actions of GnRH upon diverse ovarian functions.

Since it is unlikely that hypothalamic GnRH reaches the gonads, it is possible that the data provided here represent insight into the me-chanism of action of putative GnRH-like substances in the gonads of some species (Ying 1981). Moreover GnRH and its agonists are an ex-cellent tool for studying the biochemical events involved in oocyte maturation and induction of ovulation, two fundamental physiological processes which are not yet understood.

ACKNOWLEDGMENTS

Z.N and N.D are the incumbents of the Charles H Revson Career Devel-opment Chair and M.Z and J.M are recipients of grants-in-aid from the Chief Scientist's Bureau of the Ministry of Health, Israel.

REFERENCES

Benabe JE, Spry LA, Morrison AR (1982) Effect of angiotensin II on phosphatidylinositol and polyphosphoinosites turnover in rat kid-ney, mechanism of prostaglandin release. J Biol Chem 257:7430-7434
Clark MR (1982) Stimulation of progesterone and prostaglandin E accu-mulation by luteinizing hormone releasing hormone (LHRH) and LHRH analogs in rat granulosa cells. Endocrinology 110:146-152
Clayton RN, Harwood JP, Catt KJ (1979) Gonadotropin-releasing hormone analogue binds to luteal cells and inhibits progesterone produc-tion. Nature 282:90-92
Corbin A, Bex FJ (1981) Luteinizing hormone releasing hormone ago-nists induce ovulation in hypophysectomized proestrus rats: Direct ovarian effect. Life Sci 29:185-192
Cuatrecasas P, Hollenberg MD, Chang KJ, Bennett V (1975) Hormone re-ceptors complexes and their modulation of membrane function. Rec. Prog. Horm. Res. 31:37-94

Dekel N, Sherizly I, Tsafriri A, Naor Z (1983) A comparative study on the mechanism of action of luteinizing hormone and a gonadotropin releasing hormone analog on the ovary. Biol Reprod 28:161-166

Ekholm C, Hillensjö T, Isaksson O (1981) Gonadotropin releasing hormone agonists stimulate oocyte meiosis and ovulation in hypophysectomized rats. Endocrinology 108:2022-2024

Fain JN (1982) Involvement of phosphatidylinositol breakdown in elevation of cytosol Ca^{2+} by hormones and relationship to prostaglandin formation. In: Kohn LD (ed) Hormone Receptors, John Wiley and Sons Ltd, p. 237

Farese RV, Sabir AM (1980) Polyphosphoinositides: Stimulator of mitochondrial cholesterol side chain cleavage and possible identification as an adrenocorticotropin induced cycloheximide sensitive, cytosolic steroidogenic factor. Endocrinology 106:1869-1879

Hillensjö T, Lemaire WJ (1980) Gonadotropin releasing hormone agonists stimulate meiotic maturation of follicle-enclosed rat oocytes in vitro. Nature 287:145-146

Hokin MR, Hokin LE (1953) Enzyme secretion and the incorporation of ^{32}P into phospholipids of pancreas slices. J Biol Chem 203:967-977

Hsueh AJW, Jones PBC (1981) Extrapituitary actions of gonadotropin releasing hormone. Endocrine Reviews 2:437-461

Jones PBC, Hsueh AJW (1982) Pregnenolone biosynthesis by cultured rat granulosa cells: Modulation by follicle stimulating hormone and gonadotropin releasing hormone. Endocrinology 111:713-721

Kishimoto A, Takai Y, Mori T, Kikkawa U, Nishizuka Y (1980) Activation of calcium and phospholipid-dependent protein kinase by diacylglycerol, its possible relation to phosphatidylinositol. J Biol Chem 255:2273-2276

Knecht M, Catt KJ (1981) Gonadotropin releasing hormone: regulation of adenosine 3'5'-monophosphate in ovarian granulosa cells. Science 214:1346-1348

Knecht M, Ranta T, Naor Z, Catt KJ (1983) Direct effect of GnRH on the ovary. In: Greenwold G, Terranova P (eds) Factors regulating ovarian function. Raven Press, in press.

Lapetina EG, Billah MM, Cuatrecasas P (1981) The phosphatidylinositol cycle and the regulation of arachidonic acid production. Nature 292:367-369

Marshall PJ, Boatman DE, Hokin LE (1981) Direct demonstration of the formation of prostaglandin E$_2$ due to phosphatidylinositol breakdown associated with stimulation of enzyme secretion in the pancreas. J Biol Chem 256:844-847

Michell RH (1975) Inositol phospholipids and cell surface receptor function. Biochim Biophys Acta 415:81-147

Naor Z, Catt KJ (1981) Mechanism of action of gonadotropin releasing hormone, involvement of phospholipid turnover in luteinizing hormone release. J Biol Chem 256:2226-2229

Naor Z, Yavin E (1982) Gonadotropin releasing hormone stimulates phospholipid labeling in cultured granulosa cells. Endocrinology 111:1615-1619

Naor Z, Zilberstein M, Zakut H, Lindner HR, Dekel N (1983a) Dissociation between the direct stimulatory and inhibitory effects of a gonadotropin releasing hormone analog on ovarian functions. Mol Cell Endocrinol, in press

Naor Z, Vanderhoek JY, Lindner HR, Catt KJ (1983b) Arachidonic acid products as possible mediators of the action of gonadotropin releasing hormone. In: Samuelsson B, Paoletti R, Ramwell P (eds) Advances in prostaglandins, thromboxanes and leukotrienes research. vol 12 Raven Press. p 259-263

Putney JW, Weiss SJ, Van de Walle CM, Haddas RA (1980) Is phosphatidic acid a calcium ionophore under neurohumoral control? Nature 284:345-347

Rimon G, Hanski E, Braun S, Levitzki A (1978) Mode of coupling between hormone receptors and adenylate cyclase elucidate by modulation of membrane fluidity. Nature 276:394-396

Salmon DM, Honeyman TW (1980) Proposed mechanism of cholinergic action in smooth muscle. Nature 284:344-345

Seguin C, Belanger A, Labrie F, Hansel W (1982) Study of the direct
action of LHRH agonists at the testicular level in intact rats
treated with an anti-LH serum. Endocrinology 110:524-530

Strulovici B, Lindner HR, Shinitzky M, Zor U (1981) Elevation of apparent membrane viscosity in ovarian granulosa cells by follicle
stimulating hormone. Biochim Biophys Acta 640:159-168

Tyson CA, Zanda HV, Green DE (1976) Phospholipids as ionophores. J
Biol Chem 251:1326-1332

Ying S, Ling N, Bohlen P, Guillemin R (1981) Gonadocrinins: peptides
in ovarian follicular fluid stimulating the secretion of pituitary
gonadotropins. Endocrinology 108:1206-1215

Zilberstein M, Zakut H, Eli Y, Naor Z Regulation of prostaglandin E,
progesterone and cyclic AMP production in ovarian granulosa cells
by luteinizing hormone and gonadotropin releasing hormone agonist:
Comparative studies. Endocrinology, submitted

Zor U, Lamprecht SA, Kaneko T, Schneider HPG, McCann SM, Field JB,
Tsafriri A, Lindner HR (1972) Functional relations between cyclic
AMP, prostaglandins, and luteinizing hormone in rat pituitary and
ovary. Adv Cyc Nucl Res 1:503-520

Zor U, Lamprecht SA (1977) Mechanism of prostaglandin action in endocrine glands. In: Litwack G (ed) Biochemical actions of hormones. vol 4 Academic Press. pp 85-133

Subject Index